Pelvic Floor Exercises
for Erectile Dysfunction

Pelvic Floor Exercises for Erectile Dysfunction

Grace Dorey PhD MCSP

Visiting Senior Research Fellow, University of the West of
England, Bristol;
Physiotherapy Extended Scope Practitioner (Continence),
North Devon District Hospital, Barnstaple;
Consultant Physiotherapist (Continence), The Somerset
Nuffield Hospital, Taunton

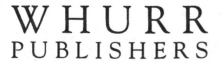

WHURR
PUBLISHERS

© 2004 Whurr Publishers Ltd
First published 2004
by Whurr Publishers Ltd
19b Compton Terrace
London N1 2UN England and
325 Chestnut Street, Philadelphia PA 19106 USA

British Library Cataloguing in Publication Data
A catalogue record for this book is available from the
British Library.

ISBN 1 86156 365 5

Typeset by Adrian McLaughlin, a@microguides.net

Contents

Foreword

As the provision of healthcare becomes more comprehensive, attention focuses increasingly on disorders that do not threaten life, yet play such a vital role in maintaining health by contributing those essential qualities of well-being or self-esteem to daily living. Erectile dysfunction and post-micturition dribble are prime examples of taboo subjects which have not attracted sufficient attention in the past, but which seriously undermine the quality of an individual's life.

In a clear, logical and scientific approach, Dr Grace Dorey has undertaken a meticulous assessment of the many factors that influence erectile function. As a physiotherapist with a special interest in continence, the complex anatomy, physiology and function of the pelvic floor muscles form the basis of this book and are described in detail, aided by simple yet fine, explicit illustrations. The bibliography is impressive and a meticulous analysis of evidence from previous studies has been included. However, the results of her personal studies with the application of a manometric biofeedback technique provide the conclusive evidence that pelvic floor exercises constitute an important therapeutic measure for men with erectile dysfunction. As if that alone is not sufficient, the author has included an additional chapter to convince the reader that physiotherapy can also cure post-micturition dribble.

Medical practice must be based on reliable evidence. Any clinician treating patients with erectile dysfunction or post-micturition dribble should read this outstanding and instructive exposition to appreciate the scientific evidence available to support the use of pelvic floor exercises as a first-line remedy.

Professor Roger Feneley
Bristol, 2003

Dedication

To the many men and their partners who have a reduced quality of life resulting from erectile difficulties.

Acknowledgements

I would like to acknowledge the dedication, guidance and support of some very special people.

I would like to thank David Butler and Adrian English, from Hollister Europe Ltd, for their generosity in kindly providing my fees at the University of the West of England, Bristol for three years.

I am truly indebted to Professor Roger Feneley, Mr Mark Speakman, Dr Margaret Miers, Professor Chris Dunn and Dr Annette Swinkels for their wisdom, commitment and diplomacy. It was a privilege to be supervised by such eminent professionals who challenged and nurtured me, but above all offered total encouragement and belief in the project.

I was privileged to have Mr Malcom Lucas as the external examiner and honoured to have Dr Kevin Foreman and Dr Richard Luxton as internal examiners. I thank them sincerely.

I am most grateful to Ginny Farnworth-Smith, Hospital Manager and to Ros Wills, Physiotherapy Manager for enabling me to conduct this research at the Somerset Nuffield Hospital, Taunton and to Angus MacCormick from the Taunton and Somerset NHST Hospital sexual dysfunction clinic for his professional collaboration.

Importantly, my thanks goes to the 55 men who participated in the trial, knowing that their attendance could improve the lives of other men similarly affected by the distress of erectile dysfunction.

Also, I would like to thank Dr Paul Ewings for providing valuable and much needed statistical help, and to Mollie Gilchrist and Dr Jon Pollock for their expertise and crisis management.

My gratitude goes to my daughter, Claire, for her accurate anatomical artwork and understanding, and my son, Martin, for his total support.

I am most grateful to Nick for his encouragement throughout my studies and for his unfailing support and belief in me during the tough times.

Finally, I would like to thank my physiotherapy colleagues who challenged my thinking, helped to develop my thought processes and who kept my feet on the ground with a mixture of experience, encouragement and humour.

Preface

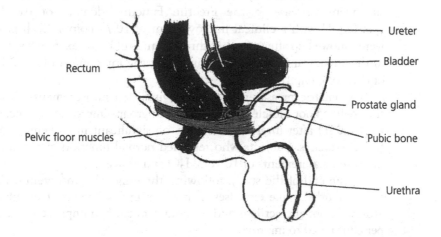

Erectile dysfunction can severely impact on the quality of life of men and their partners. The objectives of this study were to evaluate the role of pelvic floor muscle exercises and manometric biofeedback in the management of erectile dysfunction using a randomised controlled trial. Fifty-five men were randomised into two groups. Twenty-eight subjects in the intervention group received five treatments of pelvic floor muscle exercises, manometric biofeedback and lifestyle changes; 27 subjects in the control group received five sessions of lifestyle changes only. Subjects were assessed at baseline and three months. Outcome measures used were the International Index of Erectile Function, Partner's International Index of Erectile Function and Erectile Dysfunction – Effect on Quality of Life questionnaires, anal manometric measurements, digital anal grades and a blind assessment. The intervention group were followed up at a six-month assessment after a further three months of home exercises. The control group crossed over into a parallel arm after three months and received three months' intervention followed by three months of home exercises, with assessments at six and nine months.

Results from the randomised controlled part of the trial at three months showed that the subjects in the intervention group improved significantly in the Erectile Function domain of the IIEF (p = 0.001) with a clinical improvement of 6.74 points. The control group showed no significant increase in erectile function following three months of lifestyle changes only (p = 0.658). The control group then crossed over into the parallel arm and received three months of intervention. At six months, following three months of lifestyle changes and three months of the intervention, subjects in the control group showed a statistically significant increase in the Erectile Function domain of the IIEF (p < 0.001) with a clinical improvement of 10.73 points. Both groups were followed up after a further three months of home exercises with no further significant improvement in either the intervention (p = 0.108) or control group (p = 0.646).

Manometric measurements and digital anal measurements showed that pelvic floor muscle strength in both groups improved significantly (p < 0.001) after intervention, with no significant improvement after home exercises. Subjects who regained normal function attained anal pressure measurements of 100 cmH$_2$O and above.

At the end of the study, following three months' intervention and three months' home exercises in both groups, 40 per cent of subjects attained normal erectile function, 34.5 per cent had improved and 25.5 per cent failed to improve.

Post-micturition dribble was self-reported by 65.5 per cent of subjects at baseline. At the end of the trial, after intervention and home exercises in both groups, 75 per cent of subjects reported no post-micturition dribble at the blind assessment (p < 0.002).

Major findings in this study included the effectiveness of pelvic floor muscle exercises for both erectile dysfunction and post-micturition dribble, and the good reliability of anal manometric measurements to measure pelvic floor muscle strength. There was good correlation of manometric measurements with digital anal grades of pelvic floor muscle strength, but there appeared to be a need to expand the scale of digital anal grades in men. It was found that younger men performing pelvic floor muscle exercises had a better chance than older men of regaining erectile function and that men taking anti-hypertensive medication had a worse chance of regaining erectile function.

Chapter 1
Anatomy and physiology

Erectile dysfunction

Erectile dysfunction was defined by a National Institutes of Health Consensus Development Conference in 1993 as 'the inability to achieve or maintain an erection sufficient for satisfactory sexual performance (for both partners)'. The degrees of erectile dysfunction are summarised in Table 1.1.

Table 1.1: Severity of erectile dysfunction (Albaugh and Lewis, 1999)

Severity of erectile dysfunction	Satisfactory attempts out of ten
Mild	7–8
Moderate	4–6
Severe	0–3

Prevalence of erectile dysfunction

The prevalence of erectile dysfunction (ED) is unknown. Aytac et al. (1999) have estimated that 152 million men worldwide were suffering from ED in 1995, a figure projected to rise to 322 million men worldwide by 2025. However, as many as 50 per cent of men experience intermittent episodes of ED (Wagner et al., 1996; Aytac et al., 1999), although the severity is unknown; nor is it known how many men need or want treatment. Ten per cent of healthy men may be affected and significantly greater numbers of men with co-morbidities, such as hypertension (15 per cent), diabetes (28 per cent) and heart disease (39 per cent) (Feldman et al., 1994; Wagner et al., 1996). Men with erectile dysfunction may also suffer from depression and low self-esteem, and experience difficulties establishing and maintaining relationships (Hawton, 1998; Lording et al, 2000). Feldman et al. (1994) found the problem to be strongly age-related. They reported that the probable prevalence of complete or partial erectile dysfunction increased from 40 per cent in 50-year-olds to 66 per cent in 70-year-olds. However, Lewis and Mills (1999) found that age-related diseases may be the risk factors for ED rather than age itself. Thus, with increased life expectancy, the number of men with ED is predicted to increase. Society's willingness to discuss sexual matters has changed and greater public awareness of the availability of sildenafil (Viagra) and other oral therapies has resulted in more men now seeking treatment, even though products for the treatment of ED, such as vacuum pumps and penile injections, were previously available (Krane et al., 2000).

Risk factors for erectile dysfunction

There are many risk factors for erectile dysfunction. These include vascular insufficiency, hormonal abnormalities, the interruption of neural pathways as well as psychogenic factors (Table 1.2). Most patients exhibit 'mixed ED', that is, they have both organic and psychogenic factors (Stief, 2002). Some drugs contribute to the development and maintenance of ED. Lewis and Mills (1999) found 332 prescription medications to be associated with ED. These include psychotrophic drugs, cardiovascular drugs, histamine-2-receptor antagonists, hormones, anticholinergics and certain cytotoxic agents. However, the role of pharmacological agents is controversial because of the coexistence of certain pathologies or concomitant exposure to other drugs (Bortolotti et al., 1997). Erectile dysfunction is a common complication of diabetes mellitus and may affect half of diabetic men.

Other risk factors include accidental trauma, trauma from surgery and radiation therapy. Benign prostatic hyperplasia and lower urinary tract storage symptoms, particularly incontinence, are associated with erectile dysfunction, with the severity of frequency, urgency, nocturia and poor flow being significantly associated with the severity of erectile dysfunction (Baniel et al., 2000; Brookes et al., 2002).

Less well-defined risk factors, some of which are controversial, are related to lifestyle. These include smoking, high consumption of alcohol, high cholesterol levels, pelvic trauma, drug abuse and bicycling. A growing body of opinion suggests that weakness of the bulbocavernosus and ischiocavernosus muscles may be a risk factor for ED.

Treatment regimes for erectile dysfunction

Treatment regimes include oral pharmacological agents, intraurethral therapy, intracavernosal therapy, vacuum devices, androgen replacement therapy, psychotherapy and surgery (Table 1.3). The option

Table 1.2: Risk factors for erectile dysfunction

Risk factor	Possible components	Reference
Psychogenic	Marital conflict Depression Poor body image Performance-related Bereavement	Feldman et al. (1994)
Vasculogenic	Arteriogenic Venogenic	Feldman et al. (1994)
Neurogenic	Spinal cord trauma Multiple sclerosis Spinal tumours Parkinson's disease	Feldman et al. (1994)
Endocrinologic	Hormonal deficiency	Feldman et al. (1994)
Diabetic	Peripheral neuropathy Hypertension Renal failure	Benet and Melman (1995)
Drug-related	Some antihypertensives Some psychotropics Hormonal agents	Benet and Melman (1995)
Surgical trauma	Transurethral and radical prostatectomy Pelvic surgery Radiotherapy	Lewis and Mills (1999)
Lower urinary tract symptoms	Severe lower urinary tract symptoms, particularly incontinence	Frankel et al. (1998)
Prostatic	Benign prostatic hyperplasia	Baniel et al. (2000)
Lifestyle-related	Trauma to the perineum Bicycling Nicotine abuse Drug abuse Alcohol abuse	Bortolotti et al. (1997) Andersen and Bovim (1997) Rosen et al. (1991) Lewis and Mills (1999) Fabra and Porst (1999)
Weak perineal musculature	Lack of use? Ageing?	Claes and Baert (1993) Colpi et al. (1999)

chosen will depend on the assessment and advice of the clinician, the efficacy of the treatment, and patient and partner preference. Cost implications may influence treatment choice as sildenafil and apomorphine cost approximately £5–£6 a tablet.

Side-effects of treatment regimes

Oral therapy such as sildenafil is not without adverse effects (e.g. dyspepsia, headaches, visual disturbances) and is contraindicated in many men (e.g. those taking nitrates, who have had a recent stroke or myocardial infarction, or who have hypertension or hereditary degenerating retinal disorders). Largely because of cost concerns, oral therapy is prescribed in the NHS for erectile dysfunction associated with a limited number of conditions only (e.g. diabetes, post-radical prostatectomy, kidney transplant, severe distress from impotence) and to those men who received NHS-funded intracavernous and intraurethral drug therapies on 14 September 1998, the day the NHS Schedule of Limited Substances was brought into operation. Other treatment options currently available to men with erectile dysfunction are associated with similar adverse reactions and contraindications to sildenafil and/or low patient acceptance rates (e.g. topical therapies, vacuum devices, constriction bands, intraurethral drugs, intracavernous injections, penile vein surgery and penile implants) (Table 1.3). Compared with the disadvantages of current therapeutic options, conservative means such as pelvic floor muscle exercises provide a non-invasive treatment option.

Table 1.3: Relative benefits and side-effects of treatment for erectile dysfunction

Treatment	Benefits	Side-Effects	References
Lifestyle modification (reduction in alcohol and smoking, increase in fitness)	May return to normal erectile function	Nil or minimal	Bortolotti et al. (1997) Andersen and Bovim (1997) Rosen et al. (1991) Lewis and Mills (1999) Fabra and Porst (1999)
Review medication	May return to normal erectile function	Nil or minimal	Benet and Melman (1995)

Table 1.3: (contd).

Treatment	Benefits	Side-Effects	References
Oral therapy (phosphodi-esterase inhibitors type 5, nitric oxide donor and vasodilator)	Natural erection	Disturbed colour vision Dyspepsia Arthralgia Headaches Nasal congestion Possible death if taking nitrates (sildenafil) Possible arrhythmic death	Osterloh et al. (1999)
Vacuum devices	Non-invasive Inexpensive Effective in over 69 per cent of men	Psychological issues Lack of spontaneity Soft base of penis Interruption to sexual activity Cold erection Discomfort at band Trapped ejaculate	Turner et al. (1992)
Constriction bands	Easy to secure	Psychological issues Discomfort at band	Kirby et al. (1999)
Counselling/Sex therapy	May restore normal function Non-invasive Enhances rela-tionship	Nil or minimal	Daines and Barnes (1999)
Pelvic floor muscle exercises	May enhance rigidity Non-invasive	Nil or minimal	Claes and Baert (1993) Van Kampen et al. (1998)
Intracavernal injections	Rigid erection	Psychological issues Lack of spontaneity Penile nodules and fibrosis Bruising Priapism	Kirby et al. (1999)
Topical therapy	Easy to use Need condom	Penile irritation and burning	Kirby et al. (1999)
Intraurethral medications	Easy to use Need condom	Psychological issues Penile pain Bruising Priapism Fibrosis	Kirby et al. (1999)

(contd).

Table 1.3: (contd).

Treatment	Benefits	Side-Effects	References
Prosthetic implants	Easy to operate	Psychological issues May protrude in tight pants Insufficient penile girth Cold erection Unnatural intercourse Glans not filled Dyspareunia Risk of infection Device failure	Kirby et al. (1999)
Vascular surgery	Modest long term results	Psychological issues Infection Postoperative haematoma	Kirby et al. (1999)

The pelvic floor muscles

The pelvic floor muscles can be divided into a deep supportive layer, which forms the pelvic (urogenital) diaphragm and spans the opening of the bony pelvis, and a superficial layer, which is relevant to sexual function.

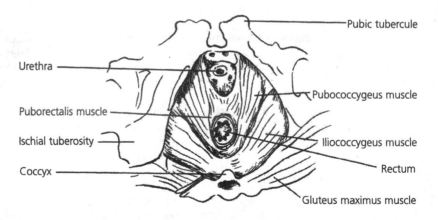

Figure 1.1: Inferior view of deep pelvic floor muscles

Deep pelvic floor muscles

The pelvic diaphragm is formed by the levator ani, which consists of the pubococcygeus muscle and the iliococcygeus muscle, together with the ischiococcygeus muscle and puborectalis muscle (Figure 1.1). The pubococcygeus muscle arises from the back of the pubic bone and the anterior part of the obturator fascia and inserts into a fibro-muscular layer between the anal canal and the coccyx. The iliococcygeus muscle arises from the ischial spine and from the arcus tendineus of the pelvic fascia and is attached to the coccyx and the median raphe. The ischiococcygeus arises from the pelvic surface of the ischial spine and is inserted into the side of the coccyx and lower sacrum. The puborectalis muscle arises from the pelvic surface of the pubic bone, blends with the levator ani and is inserted into the muscle from the other side posterior to the rectum at the anorectal flexure. It can be considered part of the pubococcygeus muscle. The external urethral sphincter lies deep to the urogenital diaphragm and surrounds the membranous urethra.

Superficial pelvic floor muscles

The anal sphincter consists of elliptical-shaped muscle fibres each side of the anal canal attached to the tip of the coccyx posteriorly and inserted into the perineal body anteriorly (Figure 1.2). Superiorly, it forms a complete sphincter and blends with the puborectalis muscle. The bulbocavernosus muscle arises from the median raphe and the perineal body. The fibres encircle the penile bulb and attach to a dorsal aponeurosis. The ischiocavernosus muscle arises from inner surface of the ischial tuberosity and the ramus of the ischium and inserts into an aponeurosis into the sides and ventral surface of the crus penis.

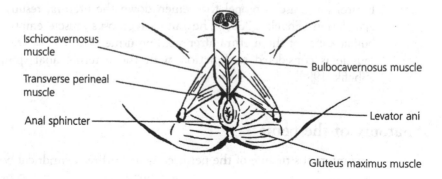

Figure 1.2: Superficial pelvic floor muscles

Nerve supply to the pelvic floor muscles

The external anal sphincter is supplied by the perineal branch of the 4th sacral nerve and by twigs from the inferior rectal branch (S2, 3) whereas the levator ani, ischicoccygeus muscle and bulbocavernosus muscle are supplied by the perineal branch of the pudendal nerve (S2, 3, 4).

Function of the pelvic floor muscles

The pelvic floor muscles have a triple function: they support the pelvic organs, maintain continence of urine and faeces, and play a role in sexual activity. The pelvic diaphragm supports the pelvic viscera and opposes the downward thrust caused by an increase in intra-abdominal pressure. The puborectalis muscle helps to maintain faecal continence by maintaining the anorectal angle. The external urethral sphincter assists in the maintenance of urinary continence, but is relaxed during micturition. The external anal sphincter is in a normal state of tonic contraction, but can provide greater occlusion of the anal aperture when needing to contain faeces and flatus. Contractions of the ischiocavernosus muscles produce an increase in the intracavernous pressure and influence penile rigidity. The area of the corpora cavernosum compressed by the ischiocavernosus muscle ranges from 35.6 per cent to 55.9 per cent (Claes et al., 1996b). The middle fibres of the bulbocavernosus muscle assist in erection of the corpus spongiosum penis by compressing the erectile tissue of the bulb of the penis. The anterior fibres spread out over the side of the corpus cavernosum and are attached to the fascia covering the dorsal vessels of the penis and contribute to erection by compressing the deep dorsal vein of the penis, thus preventing the outflow of blood from the penis. Rhythmic contractions of the bulbocavernosus muscle in conjunction with the levator ani muscles propel the semen down the urethra, resulting in ejaculation (Shafik, 2000). The bulbocavernosus muscle empties the bulbar canal of the urethra after voiding urine. The bulbocavernosus muscle is considered to function with the external anal sphincter (Shafik, 1999).

Anatomy of the penis

The internal structure of the penis consists of three cylindrical bodies: dorsally, the two corpora cavernosa communicate with each other for three-quarters of their length and ventrally the corpus spongiosum surrounds the penile portion of the urethra (Figure 1.3). The proximal end of the corpus spongiosum forms a bulb attached to the urogenital diaphragm and at the distal end expands to form the glans penis (Kirby et al., 1999). The tunica albuginea, which is composed of two layers of elastic and collagen fibres, surrounds the erectile bodies.

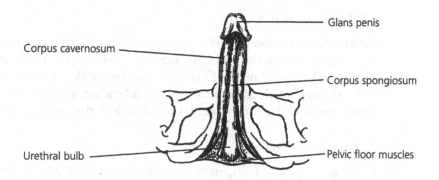

Figure 1.3: Anatomy of the penis

The erectile tissue in the corpora cavernosa and the corpus spongiosum is comprised of vascular lacunar spaces, which are surrounded by smooth muscle (Figure 1.4). The lacunar spaces derive blood from the helicine arteries, which open directly into these sinusoids. Subtunical veins between the inner and outer tunica albuginea form a network which drain blood from the erectile tissue.

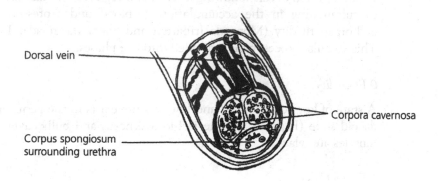

Figure 1.4: Cross-section of the penis

Physiology of penile erection

Neurophysiological classification of penile erection

From a neurophysiological aspect, erection can be classified into three types (Brock and Lue, 1993).

1 Reflexogenic erection

Reflexogenic erection originates from tactile stimulation to the genitalia. Impulses reach the spinal erection centre via sacral sensory nerves (S2–4) and thoracic nerves (T10–L2) and some follow the ascending tract culminating in sensory perception, while others activate the autonomic nuclei of the efferent nerves which induce the erection process.

2 Psychogenic erection

Psychogenic erection originates from audiovisual stimuli or fantasy. Signals descend to the spinal erection centre to activate the erection process.

3 Nocturnal erection

Nocturnal erection occurs most often during the rapid eye movement stage of sleep. Most men experience 3–5 erections lasting up to 30 minutes each in a normal night's sleep (Fisher et al., 1965). Central impulses descend the spinal cord (through an unknown mechanism) to activate the erection process.

Mechanism of erection

Penile erection occurs following a series of integrated vascular processes culminating in the accumulation of blood under pressure and end-organ rigidity (Moncada Iribarren and Sáenz de Tejada, 1999). This vascular process can be divided into five phases.

0 Flaccidity

A state of low flow of blood and low pressure exists in the penis in the flaccid state (Figure 1.5). The ischiocavernosus and bulbocavernosus muscles are relaxed.

1 Filling phase

When the erection mechanism is initiated, the parasympathetic nervous system provides excitory input to the penis from efferent segments

Flaccid state

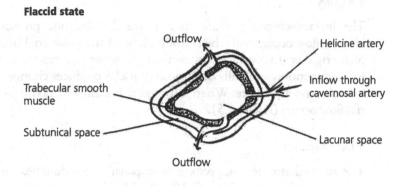

Outflow

Helicine artery

Inflow through cavernosal artery

Trabecular smooth muscle

Subtunical space

Lacunar space

Outflow

Erect state

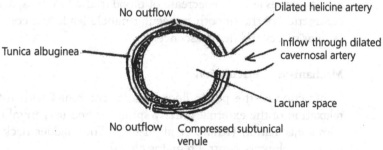

No outflow

Dilated helicine artery

Inflow through dilated cavernosal artery

Tunica albuginea

Lacunar space

No outflow   Compressed subtunical venule

Figure 1.5: Veno-occlusive mechanism of penile erection

S2–4 of the sacral spinal cord, the penile smooth arterial muscle relaxes and the cavernosal and helicine arteries dilate enabling blood to flow into the lacunar spaces.

2 Tumescence

The venous outflow is reduced by the compression of the subtunical venules against the tunica albuginea (corporal veno-occlusive mechanism) causing the penis to expand and elongate but with a scant increase in intracavernous pressure.

3 Full erection

The intracavernous pressure rapidly increases to produce full penile erection.

4 Rigidity

The intracavernous pressure rises above the diastolic pressure and blood inflow occurs with the systolic phase of the pulse enabling complete rigidity to occur. Contraction or reflex contraction of the ischiocavernosus and bulbocavernosus muscles produces changes in the intracavernous pressure. When full rigidity is achieved, no further arterial flow occurs (Figure 1.5).

5 Detumescence

The sympathetic nervous system is responsible for detumescence via thoraco-lumbar segments (T10–12, L1–2) in the spinal cord. Contraction of the smooth muscles of the penis and contraction of the penile arteries lead to a decrease of blood in the lacunar spaces and the contraction of the smooth trabecular muscle leads to a collapse of the lacunar spaces and detumescence.

Mechanism of ejaculation

Contraction of the pelvic floor muscles combined with intermittent relaxation of the external urinary sphincter and urogenital diaphragm allows ejaculation (Krane et al., 1989). The bladder neck sphincter under involuntary control remains closed.

Chapter 2
Pelvic floor exercises

Since the pioneering days of Kegel in the 1940s (Kegel, 1948), pelvic floor muscle exercises have been recognised as a first-line treatment for the restoration of bladder and bowel sphincter control and support in women (Berghmans et al., 1998). More recently, a survey has indicated that an increasing number of physiotherapists are turning their attention to the possible benefits of pelvic floor muscle exercises for the management of incontinence in men (Dorey, 2000). Pelvic floor muscle exercises appear to be effective in men suffering from incontinence after transurethral resection of the prostate (Porru et al., 2001) and following radical prostatectomy (Van Kampen et al., 2000).

Pelvic floor muscle exercises

Pelvic floor muscle exercises (PFMEs) are voluntary contractions of the pelvic floor muscles with the aim of improving their strength and endurance. During a strong pelvic floor muscle contraction, there is a visible retraction of the penis and an elevation of the testes. A pelvic floor muscle contraction evokes a reflex contraction of the cremaster muscles, which insert into the cremasteric fascia surrounding the testes. This cremasteric reflex elevates the testes. The cremaster muscle is not usually under voluntary control.

Recruitment of pelvic floor muscles

Magnetic resonance imaging (MRI) in female subjects shows that all the pelvic floor muscles contract in unison, with the coccyx moving in a ventral, cranial direction (Bø et al., 2001). The hypothesis is that a similar situation occurs in men, with the ischiocavernosus and bulbocavernosus muscles contracting along with the other pelvic floor muscles. In fact, Shafik (1999) describes the bulbocavernosus muscle as

13

part of the external anal sphincter. However, according to Lucas et al. (1999), separate components of the pelvic floor can be shown to behave independently if EMGs are recorded synchronously from different muscles. Vereecken and Verduyn (1970) used multiple EMG recordings to demonstrate desynchronisation of the levator muscles, the external urethral sphincter, the external anal sphincter and the transverse perineal muscles. This shows the importance of giving clear instructions to patients on how to achieve a penile retraction and scrotal lift, to ensure that they are voluntarily contracting the superficial pelvic floor muscles in unison with the deeper pelvic floor diaphragm.

Pelvic floor muscle strength

Each of the pelvic floor muscles is made up of approximately two-thirds type 1, slow-twitch, aerobic oxidative fibres, which are continuously tonic to support the pelvic viscera (Gosling et al., 1981). The other third are fast-twitch muscle fibres and are recruited during periods of increased intra-abdominal pressure to raise urethral closure pressure (DeLancey, 1994). When a muscle contracts, slow motor units are recruited first and, as a muscle responds to greater effort and load, the fast motor units are recruited (Jones and Round, 1990). Muscle strength development is achieved by the combination of recruitment of a greater number of motor units, a higher frequency of excitation and muscle hypertrophy (Guyton, 1986). When additional force is demanded, both slow- and fast-twitch fibres are recruited. Intensity rather than the frequency of work is important to increase muscle strength. Maximal voluntary effort is needed to address the principles of overload and specificity (DiNubile, 1991). Specificity relates to the nature of the adaptations occurring as a result of training, as all skeletal muscles have adaptive potential and can modify their structure according to demand (Bruton, 2002). High-load training leads to adaptations, which improve muscle strength, whereas repetitions or sustained contractions with low-load training leads to adaptations which improve endurance. As the strength of the muscle increases so does its surrounding capillaries, cardiovascular response and neural adaptations, thus increasing muscle endurance (Bruton, 2002). Animal studies show that hyperplasia of muscle tissue occurs during muscle training and an increase in the number of muscle fibres contributes to muscle hypertrophy (Kelley, 1996).

Pelvic floor muscle endurance

Pelvic floor muscle endurance is defined as the ability to sustain a submaximal contraction over time or the ability to perform repeated muscle contractions over time. Endurance is increased by performing a greater number of sub-maximal repetitive pelvic floor muscle contractions or by practising sustained sub-maximal muscle contractions for a longer length of time (Guyton, 1986).

Maintenance and reversibility

The optimum number of pelvic floor exercises is not known. Colpi et al. (1994) advise 30 minutes of home exercise a day, while Van Kampen et al. (1998) advise 90 contractions a day. Patient compliance may be compromised if the training sessions are too frequent or lengthy. Currently, it is not known whether pelvic floor muscle training needs to be practised daily or more/less frequently. Most trials using pelvic floor exercises have advised a daily regimen of exercises, though DiNubile (1991) suggests that strength training exercises for skeletal muscle should be practised three times a week. What is known is that if training ceases, the oxidative capacity of the muscles diminishes in 4–6 weeks, with a gradual reversion to the pre-trained state (DiNubile, 1991). With inactivity, muscle atrophy ensues, with associated loss of peak force and power (Fitts et al., 2000). However, Laycock et al. (1999) found that once an improvement is achieved, exercising maximally for one or two sessions a day may be sufficient to maintain the level of improvement. Even less exercise may be all that is needed to maintain muscle strength, provided the emphasis is placed on gaining a maximal contraction.

Functional use of pelvic floor muscles

Pelvic floor muscles need to be rehabilitated for functional demand. A 'squeeze-out' muscle contraction is a strong voluntary contraction of the pelvic floor muscles after voiding urine to eject the last few drops. It is recommended as an alternative to bulbar urethral massage for men with post-micturition dribble.

Bulbar urethral massage

Bulbar urethral massage ('urethral milking') is a self-help technique for patients suffering from post-micturition dribble. The patient is taught, after urinating, to place his fingers behind the scrotum and gently massage the bulbar urethra in a forwards and upwards direction in order to 'milk' the remaining urine from the urethra. This technique may be useful as an interim method until the pelvic floor muscles are strong enough to eject the urine from the bulbar urethra.

Sexual activity

At erection, the role of the pelvic floor muscles is to cause an increase in intracavernous pressure greater than systolic blood pressure (Lavoisier et al., 1988). Lavoisier et al. (1988) found that contractions of the pelvic floor muscles strongly coincided with changes in penile rigidity during nocturnal erections and triggered increases in intracavernous pressure to > 300 mmHg. During the thrust phase of coitus, the pelvic floor muscles and transversus abdominis muscle work synergically, aided by the larger and stronger gluteus maximus muscle. This demands optimum muscular strength and endurance and a good level of cardiovascular fitness. It is not known how much pelvic floor muscle strength and endurance are necessary to fulfil normal sexual function.

Muscles may be trained in older subjects to produce strength similar to that of a younger group (Wagner et al., 1994). A regime of daily maximal pelvic floor muscle exercises can be used to improve muscle strength, with sub-maximal work to improve muscle endurance, and may be used as a first-line treatment for erectile dysfunction. Future trials should use appropriate outcome measures.

Critical appraisal of pelvic floor muscle exercises for erectile dysfunction

Objective

The objective of the literature review was to ascertain if pelvic floor muscle exercises have merit as a conservative treatment for erectile dysfunction.

Methods

Literature search strategy

A search between 1980 and 2002 of the computerised databases Medline, AAMED (Allied and Alternative Medicine), CINAHL, EMBASE – Rehabilitation and Physical Medicine and The Cochrane Library Database was undertaken. The keywords chosen were '*erectile dysfunction, impotence, conservative treatment, physical therapy, physiotherapy, pelvic floor exercises, biofeedback, electrical stimulation* and *electrotherapy*'. A manual search was undertaken of identified manuscripts reporting research studies gained from the references in this literature.

Selection criteria

A study was included if the following criteria were addressed:
1 The trial reported the results of physiotherapy treatment for men with ED.
2 Outcome measures were reliable and relevant to the problem under investigation.

Methodological quality

Methodological rigor was assessed from a hierarchy of evidence (see Table 2.1).

Table 2.1: Levels of evidence (adapted from Sackett, 1986)

I   Strong evidence from at least one systematic review of multiple, well-designed, randomised controlled trials

II Strong evidence from at least one properly designed randomised controlled trial of appropriate size

III Evidence from well-designed trials such as non-randomised trials, cohort studies, time series or matched case-control studies

IV Evidence from well-designed non-experimental studies from more than one centre or research group

V   Opinions of respected authorities, based on the clinical evidence, descriptive studies or reports of expert committees

Each paper was assessed for the level of evidence underpinning each of the studies reviewed (Table 2.2).

Results

Included and excluded studies and levels of evidence

The literature search revealed fourteen clinical trials (Table 2.2). No level I or level II trials were found. There were eight level III trials and five level IV trials, which met the broad selection criteria and were included in this review. One trial from Russia (Karpukhin and Bogomol'nyi, 1999) revealed that the use of shock-wave massage, mud applications and local vacuum magnetotherapy stimulated coital function, but the trial was excluded due to poor methodology.

Table 2.2: Review of pelvic floor muscle exercises for erectile dysfunction

Author/design	Subjects	Method	Evidence	Outcomes
Claes & Bart (1993) Belgium *British Journal of Urology* Randomised No control	150 venous leakage ED age 23-64 median 48.7 Group 1 72 surgery Group 2 78 PFMEs	Group 1 Surgery deep dorsal vein Group 2 Information, self digital ICM 5 weekly sessions PFMEs & ICMs Home PFMEs lying, sitting & standing Digital evaluation initially 4 & 12 months with 40mg papaverine + needle EMG with maximum contraction ICMs	**Level III evidence**	Group 1 at 4 months 44 (61%) cured, 17 (23.6%) improved, 11 (15.2%) failed Group 2 at 4 months 36 (46%) cured, 22 (28%) improved, 20 (25.6%) failed Group 1 at 12 months 30 (42%) cured, 23 (32%) improved Group 2 at 12 months 33 (42%) cured, 24 (31%) improved, 45 (58%) refused surgery *Subjective outcome*
Lavoisier et al (1988) Canada *Journal of Urology* Not random No control	7 ED psychological age 28-50 mean 38.2	Recording intracavernous pressure and ICM activity with nocturnal erections Penile cuff and surface EMG over ICM	**Level IV evidence**	Over 300mmHg ischiocavernous pressure triggered by ischiocavernosus muscles *Objective outcome measured by authors*
Mamberti-Dias & Bonierbale-Branchereau (1991) France *Sexologique* Not random No control	210 ED mean age 52.5 Some venous leakage Some psychologic	PFMEs + EMG + electrical stimulation 5 - 25Hz and then 50 - 400Hz intermittent with sacral & penile or perineal electrode Visual stimulation 15 treatments	**Level III evidence**	111 (53%) cured, 44 (21%) improved, 55 (26%) failed 67% of patients attained 4/10 to 8/10 Index of Subjective Mean Rigidity *Subjective outcome*

Table 2.2: (contd).

Author/design	Subjects	Method	Evidence	Outcomes
Colpi et al 1994 Italy *Journal of Endocrinology Invest* Not random Controlled	59 ED venous leakage, age 20-63, mean 39, median 39 Group 1: 33 PFMEs + BFB Group 2: 26 controls	30 of 59 Deep dorsal vein incision 30 of 59 Psychosexual therapy No information which? Group 1 PFMEs +BFB (type unknown) Group 2 Control	**Level III evidence**	Group 1 21 (63%) out of 33 who did PFMEs cured or improved Group 2 4 (15%) out of 26 controls cured or improved 9 refused surgery *Subjective outcome*
Lavoisier et al (1986) Canada *Journal of Urology* Not random No control	9 ED (no venous leakage) age 29-65 mean 41.8	Artificial saline erection + maximal ICM contractions Needle EMG + transducer corpus cavernosum	**Level IV evidence**	ICP increases in phase with greater ICM activity Significant (p<0.01) *Objective outcome measured by authors*
Stief et al (1996) Germany *Urologe A* Not random Controlled	22 ED vasoactive non-responders	Transcutaneous electrical stimulation to smooth muscle corpus cavernosum Low frequency symmetrical trapezoidal 100-2000 µsecs, approx. 12 mA, 0.5 secs rise, 5 secs stimulation 0.5 secs rest alternating 10-20Hz and 20-35Hz	**Level IV evidence**	5 (23%) cured 3 (13.6%) responded to vaso-active drugs 14 (63.6%) failed *Subjective outcome*

(contd)

Table 2.2: (contd).

Author/design	Subjects	Method	Evidence	Outcomes
Derouet et al (1998) Germany *European Urology* Not random No control	48 ED	Transcutaneous electrical stimulation penile or perineal electrodes 20 mins daily for 3 months Bipolar, triangular Direct Current-free pulse 85μs 30Hz 3 seconds stimulation 6 seconds rest 20-120mA	**Level IV evidence**	5 (10.4%) cured 20 (41.6%) improved 23 (47.9%) failed including 10 drop outs *Subjective outcome*
Claes et al (1996b) Belgium *Journal of Urology* Not random No control	178 ED age 21-76 median 53.3	PFMEs and electrical stimulation No information on protocol	**Level III evidence**	76 (43%) cured at 4 months 55 (31%) improved 47 (26%) failed including 19 drop outs *Subjective outcome*
Van Kampen et al (1998) Belgium PhD Thesis Not random No control	51 ED various causes age 25-64 mean 46	Patient education, role of ICM & BCM. PFMEs in lying, sitting and standing + BFB anal pressure + 15 minutes electrical stimulation anal electrode or surface electrode weekly for 4 months. Symmetrical biphasic low frequency 50Hz 200μseconds, 6 seconds stimulation 12 seconds rest 90 contractions daily home exercise	**Level III evidence**	24 (46%) cured 12 (24%) improved 15 (31%) failed including 9 drop outs *Subjective outcome*

Table 2.2: (contd).

Author/design	Subjects	Method	Evidence	Outcomes
Claes et al (1995) Belgium *European Journal of Physical Medicine Rehabilitation* Not random No control	122 ED venous leakage age 21-63 median 49.5	Role of ICM & BCM + PFMEs + EMG or manometric BFB + 15 minutes electrical stimulation anal or surface electrode symmetrical biphasic low frequency 50Hz pulse 100μsecs, 6 seconds stimulation 12 seconds rest + home exercises, 40 short 50 long, evaluation initially 4 & 12 months by needle EMG of ICM	**Level III evidence**	At 4 months: 53 (43%) cured, 37 (30%) improved, 32 (26.2%) failed including 14 drop outs At 12 months 44 (36%) cured, 41 (33.6%) improved, 37 (30.3%) failed including 14 drop outs 65 (53.4%) patients refused surgery *Subjective outcome*
Schouman & Lacroix (1991) France *Ann Urologique* Not random No control	20 ED Group 1 10 venous leakage Group 2 10 psychogenic	Both groups: 10mg papaverine & electrical stimulation ICM & BCM surface electrodes + anal electrode + PFMEs + EMG BFB (position of sensors unknown), 16 sessions in 8 weeks, evaluated 6 months	**Level III evidence**	At 6 months: Group 1 6 (60%) cured or improved, 4 (40%) failed At 6 months: Group 2 5 (50%) cured or improved, 5 (50%) failed including 1 drop out *Subjective outcome*
Shafik (1996) Egypt *Andrologia* Not random No control	15 men ED age 32-55 mean 42.6	Cavernous nerve exposed through parapenile incision. Electrical stimulation 10Hz and 60Hz, bipolar platinum electrode implanted	**Level IV evidence**	Electrical stimulation at 10Hz led to tumescence and increased intracavernous pressure (P<0.01) 60Hz led to full erection *Objective outcomes by author*

(contd)

Table 2.2: (contd).

Author/design	Subjects	Method	Evidence	Outcomes
Colpi et al (1999) Italy *International J. of Impotence Research* Not random Controlled	Group 1: 76 potent men, age 18-35, mean 29.3±3.6 Group 2: 97 men with ED, age 18-35, mean 28.1±4.1 Group 3: 127 men with ED, age 36-50, mean 43.7±4.2 Group 4: 90 men with ED age 51-75, mean 58.3±5.5	Imitation of coital thrusts in side lying to increase rigidity of penis 24 maximal contractions 3 seconds hold and 6 seconds rest EMG anal probe, 2 surface electrodes on perineum and antagonists, 1 grounded electrode	**Level III evidence**	Myoelectric activity of the perineum significantly higher in potent men compared to age-matched impotent men Myoelectric activity of perineum significantly lower in men with ED over 50 years compared to younger men with ED up to 35 years and men up to 50 years *Objective outcomes by authors*

KEY:

ED   Erectile dysfunction, PFMEs Pelvic floor muscle exercises,
BCM   Bulbocavernosus muscle, ICM Ischiocavernosus muscle, BFB Biofeedback,
EMG   Electromyography, ICP Intracavernous pressure

Source of literature

Trials were conducted in Canada, Belgium, France, Germany and Italy. There were no trials from the United Kingdom.

Methodological quality and outcome of the studies

Nine trials used pelvic floor muscle exercises. Of these, three included biofeedback, one electrical stimulation, while four included biofeedback and electrical stimulation. Two trials used electrical stimulation only for ED. One trial included visual erotic stimulation (Mamberti-Dias and Bonierbale-Branchereau, 1991). Many of the studies used a small sample size and therefore provided limited evidence. Three trials (Claes and Baert, 1993; Colpi et al., 1994; Claes et al., 1995) investigated the cause of ED prior to the study. These studies considered hormonal imbalance (testosterone and prolactin), arteriogenic causes (echo doppler or arteriography), venogenic causes (dynamic caversonography and cavernometry), pharmacological evaluation (intracavernous injection of papaverine or prostaglandin E1) and nocturnal penile tumescence (Rigiscan). Rigiscan is an electronic device, designed to measure and record nocturnal penile erections. The system measures and records volumetric changes within the penis. Three electrode sets are used to monitor and record impedance data, which directly correlate to changes in penile blood volume. All patients in these trials showed a significant venous leakage on caversonography and abnormal nocturnal penile tumescence.

Clinical practice has since moved on from this rigorous testing before treatment for ED to screening for hormone imbalance due to the availability of oral medication. Schouman and Lacroix (1991) divided the sample into those men with ED due to venous leakage and those with a psychogenic cause. Van Kampen et al. (1998) classified the type of ED into five categories – venous leakage, arteriogenic, venous leakage plus arteriogenic, psychogenic and unclassified – while Colpi et al. (1999) described the aetiologic factors as psychogenic, venogenic, arteriogenic, neurogenic, fibrosis, pharmacologic, endocrine and diabetes.

Only three trials included a control group (Colpi et al., 1994; Stief et al., 1996; Colpi et al., 1999). Claes and Baert (1993) used randomisation and compared a group performing pelvic floor muscle exercises with a group undergoing surgery for erectile dysfunction.

The instructions for performing pelvic floor muscle exercises varied. In Claes and Baert (1993), patients were taught to tighten the ischiocavernosus muscle, while in the study by Schouman and Lacroix (1991) patients were taught to tighten the ischiocavernosus and bulbocavernosus muscles while achieving rigidity with 10 mg of papaverine. In Claes and Baert (1993) patients were injected with 40 mg papaverine to achieve penile rigidity and tested with needle EMG while contracting the ischiocavernosus muscle maximally.

Although Claes and Baert's (1993) work was only a level III study and lacked a control group, it was the most convincing in terms of methodology. They randomised 72 patients into a surgery group receiving excision of the deep dorsal vein and 78 patients into a pelvic floor muscle exercise group receiving five weekly sessions of patient information, pelvic floor muscle exercises and home exercises. Patients were administered 40 mg papaverine and assessed initially, at four months and at twelve months by needle electromyogram (EMG) during ischiocavernosus muscle contractions and by Rigiscan. The maximum increase in intracorporal pressure of trained subjects during muscular contractions varied between 4 and 38 per cent (median 24 per cent) at the base and between 8 and 42 per cent (median 31 per cent) at the tip of the penis. These increases in intracorporal pressure were always in phase with increases in EMG measurements of ischiocavernosus muscle activity. The EMG readings were not given.

After twelve months, patients in the pelvic floor muscle group reported a similar response (42 per cent cured and 31 per cent improved) to those in the surgery group (42 per cent cured and 32 per cent improved).

The parameters of electrical stimulation were given in six out of seven studies (Mamberti-Dias and Bonierbale-Branchereau, 1991; Claes and Baert, 1993; Claes et al., 1995; Stief et al., 1996; Derouet et al., 1998; Van Kampen et al., 1998) (Table 2.2).

The number of treatment sessions varied from 5 to 20, although some papers did not provide this information. From the available data, it appears that patients were assessed initially, and subsequently at between three and twelve months.

Discussion

Methodological limitations

The encouraging results from each of the nine studies using pelvic floor muscle exercises shows that maximal pelvic floor muscle work may aid penile rigidity and improve or even cure erectile dysfunction. However, the results should be interpreted with caution due to the poor methodology. Only one trial used randomisation; seven of the trials lacked controls; and seven provided only subjective outcomes. The lack of randomisation is an important methodological limitation, which fundamentally limited any definitive interpretation and translation of the findings from these trials.

While it is unacceptable to leave a control group without treatment, a trial could be designed to include counselling or lifestyle changes for both the treatment and the control group.

Pelvic floor muscle exercises

In four trials (Schouman and Lacroix, 1991; Claes and Baert, 1993; Claes et al., 1995; Van Kampen et al., 1998) men were encouraged to perform specific ischiocavernosus muscle and bulbocavernosus muscle exercises rather than pelvic floor muscle exercises alone. In another four studies (Lavoisier et al., 1986; Wespes et al., 1990; Schouman and Lacroix, 1991; Colpi et al., 1999) men performed ischiocavernosus muscle and bulbocavernosus muscle exercises with an erect penis, which demonstrated the need to exercise the specific muscles concerned with penile rigidity. Lavoisier et al. (1986) showed that patients with ED but without venous occlusive dysfunction gained increased intracavernous pressure when asked to perform maximal voluntary contractions of ischiocavernosus muscles with an artificially induced erection. They stated that this increase in intracavernous pressure would not have occurred if the cavernosous cavities were not completely engorged. This research indicates that men should be advised to use these muscles during coitus. Colpi et al. (1999) monitored the strength of the perineal muscles by EMG in right side lying with the subjects simulating coital thrusts. They found that pelvic floor muscle activity was significantly higher in potent men than age-matched impotent men and that in impotent men aged over 51 years pelvic floor muscle efficiency was significantly reduced. They concluded that ageing may affect voluntary contractile capacity because of the tendency to a more sedentary lifestyle and to systemic pathologies, such as diabetes, liver dysfunction, arteriosclerosis and neuropathies, which may cause decreases in muscle mass. Pelvic floor exercises could be used to prevent or reverse muscle weakness caused by disuse and may delay the onset of some pathologies.

If the activity of the ischiocavernosus muscles increases penile rigidity, then weak musculature, associated with ageing, might reasonably be expected to produce a decrease in penile rigidity and reduced erectile function. This was suggested by Colpi et al. (1999), who demonstrated with anal and perineal EMG that pelvic floor muscle efficiency was decreased in patients suffering from ED, particularly in older men. However, this may have been due to the length of time the older group had experienced ED. Claes and Baert (1993) did not report EMG or digital evaluation measurements of ischiocavernosus muscle activity during initial and follow-up assessments. Had they done so, it might have added weight to Colpi et al.'s (1999) findings.

Mamberti-Dias et al. (1999) argue that there must be an ischiocavernosus reflex similar to the bulbocavernosus reflex (pressure on the glans penis elicits a contraction of the bulbocavernosus muscles in a neurologically intact man) which can be triggered by a variation of pressure from 20 to 40 mmHg on the glans penis. Similarly, Lavoisier et al. (1992) hypothesised that, during coitus, the glans penis is subjected to varying amounts of phasic pressure stimulation which elicits reflex contractions of the ischiocavernosus muscles and increased penile rigidity.

Patient position

Another methodological limitation was the position chosen for pelvic floor muscle exercises. Colpi et al. (1999) used side lying for coital thrust simulation, while Van Kampen et al. (1998) used three positions: supine lying with knees bent and feet on the couch; sitting; and standing. It is difficult to compare trials with exercises performed in different positions, some of which may be different from the functional positions of coitus. Another difficulty for the patient is the ability to exercise in a clinical setting. They may find it embarrassing and not conducive to a good performance.

Psychosexual issues

All the trials used heterosexual men. No study mentioned any cultural factors. Perceptions of sexual activity vary from one man to another and impact on the expectations and subjective measurement of sexual performance. Not all men wish to practise penetrative sex. There were no studies that identified and addressed the difficulties and needs of homosexual men who practised anal intercourse. These factors underpin issues in the counselling of patients with ED.

Source of literature

The lack of UK trials using pelvic floor muscle exercises for erectile dysfunction was one reason why the subject was explored in this study. It may have been that health professionals in the UK were unwilling to explore this area due to embarrassment, lack of training or a belief that psychogenic factors, such as unresponsiveness, inhibition or partner- and performance-related issues, played a strong role. Therapists' perception of psychogenic factors in the UK may be different from those of therapists from other cultures. UK therapists may consider the cause of ED to be more psychological than organic and therefore leave the treatment of these men to psychologists, sexual therapists and counsellors.

Patient information

Only three trials (Claes and Baert, 1993; Claes et al., 1996b; Van Kampen et al., 1998) included patient education. This focused on pelvic anatomy and the function of the ischiocavernosus and bulbo-cavernosus muscles. Colpi et al. (1994) expected men to perform exercises at home for 30 minutes a day for nine months as a realistic alternative to surgery. No trial mentioned long-term follow-up or advised a maintenance programme for life, although Claes and Baert (1993) and Claes et al. (1995) followed up subjects for twelve months and found encouraging results.

Advice

Only one study specified the advice given to patients. Mamberti-Dias and Bonierbale-Branchereau (1991) gave advice concerning visual erotic stimulation and fantasy. Men whose ED has a psychological cause may benefit from sex therapy; though all patients might benefit from this form of treatment. For men suffering from ED due to organic causes may have a psychosomatic overlay due to performance anxiety and the accompanying psychological stress.

Intracavernous pressure

Lavoisier et al. (1986) and Wespes et al. (1990) demonstrated an increase in intracavernous pressure during contractions of the ischio-cavernosus muscle and bulbocavernosus muscle in men with ED. Lavoisier et al. (1986) showed an increase of between 100 mmHg and 525 mmHg (average 298 mmHg) ($p < 0.01$), while Michal et al. (1983) demonstrated an increase in the intracavernous pressure of the tumes-cent penis by at least 100 mmHg by pelvic floor contractions in healthy men. These three trials were undertaken under laboratory conditions. Meehan and Goldstein (1983) showed that during masturbation intra-cavernous pressure increased to ten times the arterial blood pressure. The ischiocavernosus muscle has clearly been shown to have a role in increasing the pressure in the tumescent penis. This supports the work done by Claes et al. (1996a), who dissected the corpora cavernosa of 30 male cadavers and found that 35.6–55.9 per cent of the area of the cor-pora cavernosum was compressed by the ischiocavernosus muscle.

Objective outcomes

Using anal plug electromyography as an objective outcome measure, Colpi et al. (1999) studied the contractile activity of the perineal mus-cles of 76 sexually potent men aged between 18 and 35 years and 97 age-matched impotent men. A further 217 older impotent men aged 36–75 years were studied to verify the impact of age on the efficiency of perineal floor contraction. Myoelectric activity was significantly higher in sexually potent young men (20.3 μV ± 6.2) in comparison to impotent young men (16.8 μV ± 7.2) (p = 0.0007) and significantly higher in younger impotent men than in older impotent men (13.5 μV ± 6.0) (p = 0.0009). The results showed that perineal contraction was significantly higher (p = 0.0007) in potent than in impotent men. In addition, in older impotent men perineal floor efficiency was negatively correlated to age (r = –0.21, p = 0.002). The authors reported that these results supported the hypothesis that pelvic floor efficiency may be related to erectile dysfunction and that the reinforcement of the striated muscles of the penis achieved through physiotherapy, directly or indirectly, may improve penile erection. In this trial there was no control group and the reduction in EMG activity in the pelvic floor muscles in impotent elderly men may have been due to a progression of ED or concomitant pathologies, and not age.

Lavoisier et al. (1986) and Wespes et al. (1990) used a pressure transducer as an invasive outcome method of measuring ischiocavernous pressure. Lavoisier et al. (1988) used a non-invasive penile cuff (Medasonic) made of non-elastic material filled with water. The pressure of the water correlated with ischiocavernous pressure (p > 0.001). Mamberti-Dias et al. (1999) measured the pubo-anal distance to ascertain whether an elongated bulbocavernosus muscle was a risk factor for ED, but their results were inconclusive.

Subjective outcomes

No studies used the subjective (completed by the subject) validated International Index of Erectile Function (IIEF) questionnaire as an outcome measure (Rosen et al., 1997).

Mamberti-Dias and Bonierbale-Branchereau (1991) used an index of subjective mean rigidity (ISMR) as one of the outcome measures in a non-randomised, uncontrolled study using pelvic floor exercises, EMG biofeedback and electrical stimulation of 210 men with ED. They reported an increase from 4 out of 10 to 8 out of 10 mean ISMR.

Most outcomes used patient-reported 'cure', 'improved' or 'failure'. 'Cure' was defined as an erection suitable for satisfactory sexual performance with vaginal penetration in all studies. 'Improvement' was defined in a number of ways from 'a significant increase of erection quality and performance' (Colpi et al., 1994) to 'partial response for those patients who reported some increase in quality (duration or rigidity) of erections but not sufficient for sexual intercourse' (Claes et al., 1995). No study independently verified the outcome of treatment from the partner.

Inclusion of the partner in the diagnostic process might have changed the clinical picture and the treatment recommendations (Beutel, 1999); it might also have produced outcomes with greater reliability. However, the use of the Rigiscan before and after treatment would have provided a more objective outcome measure.

Quality of life evaluation

Van Kampen et al. (1998) added a quality of life evaluation in relation to sexual function in patients at one, six, twelve and fifteen months after radical prostatectomy. They used a self-administered questionnaire with a seven-point score under the headings 'excellent', 'satisfied', 'content', 'indifferent', 'pity', 'unhappy' and 'unacceptable' in order to gain qualitative outcomes. Since this trial, the Erectile Dysfunction-Effect on Quality of Life (ED-EQoL) has been extensively tested and validated. This might have provided more rigorous data (MacDonagh et al., 2002).

Pelvic floor muscle exercises with biofeedback

Five trials used pelvic floor muscle exercises with biofeedback to provide patient awareness and stimulate increased effort. Of these, two (Colpi et al., 1994; 1999) included biofeedback as the only other modality, while three (Schouman and Lacroix, 1991; Claes et al., 1995; Van Kampen et al., 1998) combined pelvic floor muscle exercises with biofeedback and electrical stimulation. Similar techniques have been used to treat urinary and faecal incontinence and other pelvic muscle dysfunctions (La Pera and Nicastro, 1996; Ballard, 1997; Mamberti-Dias et al., 1999). It is impossible to determine which modality has caused the effect when three modalities are used.

La Pera and Nicastro (1996) used pelvic floor muscle exercises, pressure biofeedback and electrical stimulation in a non-randomised and non-controlled trial of 18 patients (age range 20–52 years) to treat premature ejaculation. The results showed that eleven patients (61 per cent) were cured associated with improved pelvic floor muscle control. Lombardi (1999) used electrical stimulation alternated with biofeedback for premature ejaculation (details unknown).

Although some trials used needle EMG and some preferred to use surface or anal EMG, others used anal manometry. Anal manometry and anal EMG monitor the pelvic floor muscles but perineal EMG and needle EMG target the ischiocavernosus muscles, the muscles demonstrated to increase intracavernous pressure and therefore increase penile rigidity.

Electrical stimulation for the treatment of erectile dysfunction

In the absence of appropriate controls, when electrical stimulation is combined with pelvic floor muscle exercises, it is impossible to determine which modality has produced the effect. However, two trials used electrical stimulation alone. Derouet et al. (1998) found electrical stimulation to the ischiocavernosus muscle produced only a 10.4 per cent cure rate, while in a controlled trial Stief et al. (1996) explored transcutaneous electrical stimulation to the smooth muscle of the penile corpus cavernosum and effected a 23 per cent cure rate. In the Derouet et al. (1998) trial, the pulse protocol and parameters were designed for striated muscle, but there may have been simultaneous stimulation of cavernosal smooth muscle tissue due to the use of penile electrodes. Whatever effect was achieved, both cure rates were low compared to the pelvic floor muscle exercise trials. This endorses the work undertaken by Berghmans et al. (1998), who systematically reviewed treatment for female stress incontinence and concluded that electrical stimulation may be no more effective than pelvic floor muscle exercises alone, but may be particularly appropriate to initiate a muscle contraction.

Conservative management for the prevention of erectile dysfunction

No publications were found describing the use of preventive conservative treatment. But if the pelvic floor musculature is poor and pelvic floor muscle exercises can be demonstrated to relieve ED, it seems reasonable to suppose that preventative muscle strengthening may help to prevent ED.

Conclusions

There is grade III level evidence that the ischiocavernosus and bulbocavernosus muscles increase penile rigidity in the tumescent penis. It is suggested that pelvic floor muscle efficiency is higher in potent than impotent men and that perineal muscle efficiency declines with age in impotent men. From the literature review, pelvic floor muscle exercises using the ischiocavernosus and bulbocavernosus muscles seem to have merit as a treatment for erectile dysfunction due to mild or moderate venous leakage and appear to be a realistic alternative to surgery. Men suffering from erectile dysfunction due to other causes may also benefit. Patients suffering from urinary incontinence and post-micturition dribble could combine a simultaneous training programme of pelvic floor muscle exercises. For those patients who appear to have been cured or improved with pelvic floor muscle exercises, it may be prudent to continue these simple exercises for life to avoid a return of ED or surgery.

Thus, the age-old adage 'use it or lose it' may well apply to the pelvic floor musculature.

Compliance may be a problem for men advised to perform daily pelvic floor muscle exercises for 30 minutes a day, or to perform 90 contractions a day, or those who are instructed to exercise 'every hour on the hour'. Following initial pelvic floor training for strength and endurance, it may be possible to maintain muscle performance with a minimal exercise programme.

There was no strong evidence that electrical stimulation was effective. No studies demonstrating preventative conservative treatment were found.

Randomised controlled trials with larger sample numbers are needed to explore the use of pelvic floor exercises as a first-line treatment for men with erectile dysfunction. Similar trials are needed to ascertain the role of pelvic floor exercises as prophylaxis for erectile dysfunction.

Outcome measures

Objectives

A literature review was undertaken, in order to select appropriate outcome measures to study the efficacy of pelvic floor muscle exercises for erectile dyfunction.

Methods

Literature search strategy

A search from the following computerised databases from 1980 to 2002 was undertaken: Medline, AAMED (Allied and Alternative Medicine), CINAHL, Nursing Collection, EMBASE – Rehabilitation and Physical Medicine and The Cochrane Library Database. The keywords chosen were 'outcome measures, assessments, questionnaires, erectile dysfunction, sexual dysfunction, impotence, erectile function, sexual function, physical therapy, physiotherapy, pelvic floor muscle exercises, biofeedback, electromyography, manometric, electrical stimulation, electrotherapy, acupuncture, conservative treatment and quality of life'. A manual search was undertaken of manuscripts found from the references of this literature.

Inclusion criteria

Any paper that used an outcome measure to test the effectiveness of conservative treatment for ED was included in the review.

Exclusion criteria

Papers that used outcome measures for the assessment of conditions other than ED and papers that measured outcome from surgery were excluded.

Results

Table 2.3: Outcome measures for erectile dysfunction

Outcome Measure	Type	Validity	Reliability and Responsiveness
IIEF	Subjective questionnaire	Validated in 10 languages	High reliability α 0.73–0.91 p < 0.0001
IIEF-5	Subjective questionnaire	Validated in 30 languages	Correlated well with IIEF Treatment changes 0.73
Patient EDITS	Subjective questionnaire	Good content validity	Internal consistency 0.90 Reliability 0.98
Partner EDITS	Subjective questionnaire	Good content validity	Internal consistency 0.76 Reliability 0.83
ICSsex	Subjective questionnaire	Good content and validity	Used with validated ICSmale and ICSQoL
PROTOsex	Subjective questionnaire	Updated version of ICSsex	
QOL-MED	Subjective questionnaire	Not validated	Qualitative data scored quantitatively
ED-EQoL	Subjective questionnaire	Good face and content validity	α 0.94 Responsive to change
Veterans Affairs Questionnaire	Subjective questionnaire	Preliminary validation	Internal consistency α 0.54–0.82
RSSF	Subjective questionnaire	Good content validity	High reliability 90 per cent
Brief Sexual Function Inventory	Subjective questionnaire		Internal consistency α 0.81 Reliability r = 0.87
CMSH-SFQ	Subjective questionnaire	Acceptable validity	Acceptable reliability p < 0.001

Table 2.3: (contd).

Outcome Measure	Type	Validity	Reliability and Responsiveness
Likert scale	Subjective	Categorical data	
Visual analogue scale	Subjective/ Objective	Interval data	
Clinician's questions	Subjective	Nominal and categorical data	
Patients' set goals	Subjective	Measured qualitatively	
Radial rigidity	Objective		r > 0.80 (10 per cent erection)
Snap Gauge band	Objective	Compared well with volume phallometry > 2.5 mm Pearson correlations (r > 0.80) correlated well with Rigiscan	
Axial rigidity	Objective	Measure of penile shaft buckling to downward force of 1 kg	
Colour duplex Doppler	Objective	Measure of changes in cavernous diameter and arterial flow	
Pudendal nerve conduction test	Objective	Measure of nerve conductivity	
Intra-cavernous pressure	Objective	Invasive or non-invasive measure Non-invasive p < 0.001	
Ischiocavernosus muscle power	Objective	Measure of muscle contraction distance, endurance and power	
EMG	Objective	Interval/ratio data in µV	
Manometry	Objective	Interval/ratio data in mmHg or cmH_2O	
Digital anal examination	Objective	Interval data on 0–5 scale	
Clinician's assessment	Objective	Categorical data	

LUTS	Lower urinary tract symptoms	ED-EQoL	Erectile Dysfunction – Effect on Quality of Life
IIEF	International Index of Erectile Function	QOL-MED	Quality of Life – Measure for Erectile Dysfunction Questionnaire
IIEF-5	International Index of Erectile Function - 5	RSSF	Radiumhemmets Scale of Sexual Function
EDITS	Erectile Dysfunction Inventory of Treatment Satisfaction	VAQ	Veterans' Affairs Questionnaire
ICSsex	International Continence Society sex questionnaire	BSFI	Brief Sexual Function Inventory
PROTOsex	PROstate Trials Office sex instrument	CMSH-SFQ	Centre for Marital and Sexual Health-Sexual Functioning Questionnaire

Of a total of 27 outcome measures found for ED, 15 were subjective (patient- or partner-reported) and twelve objective (measured by a clinician) (Table 2.3). Ten subjective questionnaires were found which have been used as outcome measures for men with ED and only one was found for partners. One validated (ED-EQoL) and one unvalidated (QOL-MED) questionnaire specifically addressed quality of life in men. Questionnaires addressed or placed emphasis on different components of erectile dysfunction. The domains addressed are listed in Table 2.4.

Table 2.4: Question categories of questionnaires assessing male sexual function

	IIEF	IIEF-5	EDITS	ICS sex	PRO TOsex	ED-EQoL	QOL -MED	RSSF	VAQ	BSFI	CMSH-SFQ
Rigidity of erections	6	5		1	1		1	7		4	1
Psychological aspect						13	12				
Orgasmic function	1							4		3	1
Sexual desire	2						1	2		3	1
Intercourse satisfaction	3			1	1		1	2	1		1
Ejaculation	1			1	2			3			
LUTS impact on sex life				1	1				1		
Sexual relationship	1				1		10				
Overall satisfaction			11					2		1	1
Partner satisfaction			5			2					
Social activity							1		2		
Quality of life	1						1		1		
Total questions	15	5	16	4	6	15	27	20	5	11	5

Key:

LUTS	Lower urinary tract symptoms
IIEF	International Index of Erectile Function
IIEF-5	International Index of Erectile Function - 5
EDITS	Erectile Dysfunction Inventory of Treatment Satisfaction
ICSsex	International Continence Society sex questionnaire
PROTOsex	PROstate Trials Office sex instrument
ED-EQol	Erectile Dysfunction – Effect on Quality of Life
QOL-MED	Quality of Life – Measure for Erectile Dysfunction Questionnaire
RSSF	Radiumhemmets Scale of Sexual Satisfaction
VAQ	Veterans' Affairs Questionnaire
BSFI	Brief Sexual Function Inventory
CMSH-SFQ	Centre for Marital and Sexual Health – Sexual Functioning Questionnaire

Discussion

Subjective outcome measures

The use of subjective questionnaires providing symptom scales and quality of life measures can assist the clinician in obtaining data in a standardised, cost-efficient and sensitive manner. The difficulty with ED is that it is a self-reported condition with no objective diagnostic tests available for its confirmation (Rosen et al., 1999a). In the clinical setting, questionnaires can be used to complement, not replace, a full clinical assessment, including a medical history of at least six months' duration and a physical examination (Cappelleri and Rosen, 1999). Limitations of the fifteen questions of the IIEF instrument are the fact that it does not address non-erectile components of sexual response and partner relationship. In fact, no questionnaire followed the recommendations of the First International Consultation on Erectile Dysfunction and addressed specific religious, cultural, educational and economic factors of the individual patient (Recommendations of the First International Consultation on Erectile Dysfunction, 2000). These recommendations stated that assessment should include identification of patient needs, expectations, priorities and treatment preferences, which may be significantly influenced by cultural, social, ethnic and religious perspectives.

In clinical trials, standardisation is necessary to compare one trial with another. When determining benefit and risk, both pre- and post-treatment assessments need to be standardised, validated and accepted by the scientific community (Wyllie, 2000). The IIEF is a valid, reliable and responsive instrument, which has been used widely for drug trials. An increase of six points in the erectile function domain of the IIEF was considered clinically significant and shifted the score into another category (Goldstein, 2000) (Table 2.5).

Table 2.5: Erectile function domain categories of IIEF (Goldstein, 2000)

Erectile Function Domain Category	Score
Severe erectile dysfunction	0–6
Moderate–severe erectile dysfunction	7–12
Moderate erectile dysfunction	13–18
Mild erectile dysfunction	19–24
Normal erectile function	25–30

The advent of the IIEF-5 provided a valid measurement tool, which was more patient-friendly. The IIEF-5 used five items from the IIEF six-item erectile function domain, whereas the IIEF was designed for clinical trials and not well suited as a simple screening measure to supplement physical examination and medical history in the clinical setting. However, the IIEF-5 was designed to enhance a clinical assessment and provide information regarding symptom severity and impact rather than to replace the IIEF for drug trials. Neither the IIEF nor IIEF-5 was suitable for population-based studies where detailed clinical measures of ED were impractical. In this situation a single question as in the Male Massachusetts Aging Study (MMAS) was found to be a practical tool (Feldman et al., 1994).

Even researchers using the IIEF lacked of standardisation in analysis. In their trial, Rosen et al. (1997) analysed all the IIEF questions. Some trials reported each domain separately (Lowentritt et al., 1999; Goldstein, 2000), some used just the erectile function domain, while others highlighted only question 3 ('*Over the past four weeks, when you attempted sexual intercourse, how often were you able to penetrate your partner?*') and question 4 ('*Over the past four weeks, during sexual intercourse, how often were you able to maintain your erection after you had penetrated you partner?*') (Rendell et al., 1999; Blander et al., 2000). However, researchers investigating sexual dysfunction in men with lower urinary tract symptoms used a different set of questions from the ICS*sex* questionnaire as part of the ICS*male* questionnaire (Frankel et al., 1998).

The IIEF asks questions concerning the last month's sexual activity, while the IIEF-5 addresses the previous three months' sexual activity, or the last time sexual activity took place. This is linked to the consistency element of the definition of erectile dysfunction where a three-month minimum duration is generally accepted (Recommendations of the First International Consultation on Erectile Dysfunction, 2000). However, Rosen et al. (1999a) referred to a six-month period for IIEF-5 questions.

One of the problems with the IIEF is the difficulty of assessing men who do not have a partner or do not have sexual intercourse with their partner, or have sexual contact but not intercourse (Cappelleri and Rosen, 1999).

Surprisingly, the search revealed only one partner's questionnaire: the partner's Erectile Dysfunction Inventory of Treatment Satisfaction (EDITS). Partner involvement is becoming increasingly recognised in the treatment of ED (Dorey, 2001a). The partner's cultural and social preferences should be considered. EDITS was developed to assess both the patient's and their partner's satisfaction with medical treatments for ED (Althof et al., 1999). Only two studies (Aydin et al., 1997; Kho et al, 1999) used a method of obtaining independent verification from the partner as to the outcome of treatment. Collection of such data may have produced more meaningful outcomes.

Only two quality of life instruments (QOL-MED and ED-EQoL) were found (Wagner et al., 1996; MacDonagh et al., 2002). The unvalidated QOL-MED has been superseded by the ED-EQoL, which has been recently validated. There are limitations to both quality of life questionnaires. There are fifteen questions, which are time-consuming to complete, particularly when combined with an erectile function questionnaire such as the IIEF. Also, they fail to address cultural issues and pose a need for a validated cross-cultural quality of life measure. Other questionnaires included a single general quality of life question. For clinical trials one question may not suffice and a quality of life instrument would provide subtler information in this important area.

Subjective questionnaires such as the IIEF use a five-point Likert scale from 'Almost always' to 'Almost never' to monitor categorical data (Likert, 1952) (Appendix 1). Other subjective measures, such as clinician's questions, provide a nominal level of data with only a basic level of information (Hicks, 1995).

Objective outcome measures

There is an increasing tendency to use pharmaco-testing with sub-lingual apomorphine or sildenafil in preliminary diagnostic testing for erectile dysfunction (Wagner et al., 2002).

Pelvic floor muscle strength can be measured using digital anal examination, anal manometry, and anal or surface EMG. Digital anal examination has been found to be a valid and reliable method of assessing puborectalis muscle strength in men when performed by an experienced investigator (Wyndaele and Van Eetvelde, 1996). Each subject was positioned in supine lying with knees bent and apart and feet placed on the bed, and the examining finger introduced 3–4 cm from the anal meatus to palpate the puborectalis muscle at the ano-rectal angle (Laycock, 1994a). These muscles could be graded, as for any voluntary muscle in the body, on a scale of 0–5 for muscle strength using the modified Oxford scale, for the duration of hold and for the ability to perform fast contractions (Laycock, 1994b) (Table 2.6).

Table 2.6: Assessment of strength of the pelvic floor muscles (Laycock, 1994b)

Description	Grade
Nil	0
Flicker	1
Weak	2
Moderate	3
Good	4
Strong	5

Wyndaele and Van Eetvelde (1996) found digital anal examination to be a more reproducible technique than surface palpation of the more superficial bulbocavernosus muscle. In contrast to the ease of tightening of the external anal sphincter, some difficulty in isolating and performing a bulbocavernosus muscle contraction in healthy young men was reported. However, the external anal sphincter is an integral part of the bulbocavernosus muscle (Shafik, 1999) and therefore digital anal examination could test the combined strength of these muscles. Despite its reliability, digital anal examination has a number of limitations: it provides only ordinal data, requires a skilled clinician and visual feedback to the patient is absent.

Anal manometry with an air-filled pressure probe has previously been used to monitor the strength of pelvic floor muscles for men with urinary incontinence (Burgio et al., 1989). Dorey and Swinkels (2002) found manometric measurements with an anal pressure probe to have good within-day and day-to-day reliability. Anal manometry in cmH_2O assessed the squeeze pressure of the puborectalis muscle reinforced by external anal sphincter and the pelvic floor musculature.

Electromyography to the ischiocavernosus was performed using needle EMG (Claes and Baert, 1993) or EMG with an anal probe (Van Kampen et al., 2000). Electromyography is a method of recording and quantifying the electrical activity produced by the muscle fibres of activated motor units (Sale, 1992). The EMG signal is not a true measurement of muscle strength but an indication of the bioelectrical activity in the muscle (Vodušek, 1994). Therefore, after strength training, it is not possible to infer that the force produced is greater if EMG activity is increased (Clarys and Cabri, 1993). In addition, during EMG biofeedback, the signal or noise from larger muscle groups may be picked up (Herrington, 1996). EMG may be used to measure pelvic floor muscle activity using a needle probe, surface electrodes or anal probe. However, these methods have some drawbacks. According to Vereecken et al. (1982), the EMG spectrum is influenced by a number of factors. These include the type of electrode, its distance from the muscle fibre, the diameter of the single fibres, the number of muscle fibres within the motor unit and the architecture within the motor unit. A needle probe is invasive, detects activity from few motor fibres and poses problems with accurate electrode placement (Berger, 1995). Similarly, electrode placement problems affect the reproducibility and accuracy of EMG recordings taken from both surface and anal electrodes (Haslam, 1999) although anal EMG probes make closer contact with the puborectalis muscle. Haslam (1999) found good correlation between vaginal EMG, vaginal manometry and digital vaginal examination in women (p < 0.05), though it remains unknown in men or women anally.

Both anal manometry and electromyography monitor the activity of the external anal sphincter and the puborectalis muscle. However, international standardisation is needed for manometric equipment which currently measures pressure in cmH_2O (Carapeti et al., 1999; Savoye et al., 2000), mmHg (Glia et al., 1997; Fynes et al., 1999) or millibars (Marzio et al., 1998). Van Kampen et al. (2000) and Moore et al. (1999) used a digital anal examination with a modified Oxford scale (0–5) as an outcome measure to assess the strength and endurance (0–10 seconds) of the pelvic floor muscles following radical prostatectomy. However, other clinical trials have graded pelvic floor muscles 0–3 (Jackson et al., 1996) and 0–4 (Paterson et al., 1997; Chang et al., 1998). It would be reasonable to suggest the merit of having an internationally recommended scoring system in order to make comparisons between studies more meaningful.

The improvement in strength, endurance and activity of the pelvic floor muscles can be monitored by various outcome measures. Pudendal nerve conduction tests show whether the nerve to the pelvic floor musculature is compromised. Outcome measures for pelvic floor muscle strength can be rather unsophisticated. The maximum strength and endurance of the ischiocavernosus muscle and the distance shortened were evaluated with a spring balance attached to the glans penis (Kawanishi et al., 2000). The patient was supine, with one end of the spring balance strapped to the glans penis and the other end fixed to a support above his head. Maximum contractile power in unaffected men was more than two and a half times greater than men with venogenic ED.

A visual analogue scale can be useful to assess qualitative data, such as the 'quality of life' or 'bother', in a quantitative way, for each symptom. If the unmarked 10 cm line is subsequently measured, visual analogue data may be treated objectively as interval/ratio (Hicks, 1995).

The most widely used objective measure of penile engorgement is Rigiscan, which can distinguish between organic and psychogenic erectile dysfunction. It is more sophisticated than a clinical estimation of erection on a 0 (no response) to 5 (full rigidity) scale (Kunelius and Lukkarinen, 1999) and is used widely in research. The major limitation of radial rigidity measurement is the assumption that there is a correlation between radial and axial rigidity (Wyllie, 2000), although studies have confirmed a relationship between radial compressibility, intracorporal pressure and axial buckling force (Frohrib et al., 1987).

Axial rigidity monitoring was originally performed in the unnatural setting of a sleep laboratory. This was superseded by nocturnal penile tumescence and rigidity monitoring at home. Udelson et al. (1999) showed that axial and radial rigidity have a common dependency on intracavernosal pressure. However, radial rigidity values varied with tunical surface wall tension forces and reached a maximum finite value, whereas axial rigidity values increased towards infinity. They suggested that axial and not radial rigidity should be measured to assess functional penile rigidity. However, Timm (1999) argues that axial penile buckling is unreliable, invasive and operator-dependent, has greatly limited reproducibility and may damage the thin-walled pressurised penile vessels. In fact, there are many factors other than radial and axial rigidity, such as Peyronie's disease, vaginal size, lubrication and partner receptivity, that make intromission vary.

Colour Duplex Doppler Ultrasound reveals penile anatomy as well as haemodynamics. It is particularly useful in providing vascular profiles of the reasons why some men are oral agent-resistant (Broderick, 1999). However, Slob et al. (2002) revealed that colour Doppler sonography often resulted in incorrect diagnosis by presuming a vascular abnormality.

From this literature review, it can be seen that different outcome measures are needed for each of the separate components of ED (Table 2.7). It is recommended that outcome instruments should be carefully selected to provide the best possible scientific data in terms of the levels of validity, reliability and responsiveness.

Table 2.7: Recommended outcome measures for each component of erectile dysfunction

Erectile Dysfunction Component	Outcome Measure	
	Subjective	Objective
Rigidity	IIEF IIEF-5	Radial rigidity Snap gauge band
Vascular flow		Colour Duplex Doppler
Nerve conductivity		Pudendal nerve conduction
Intra-cavernosal pressure		Pressure transducer Penile cuff
Pelvic floor muscle activity		Needle EMG Anal EMG Surface EMG Anal manometry Digital anal
Partner satisfaction	Partner Erectile Dysfunction Inventory of Treatment Satisfaction	
Quality of life	ED-EQoL	

Lifestyle risk factors for erectile dysfunction

Various lifestyle risk factors, either singly or together, may have a dele-
terious effect on erectile function. These include smoking, a high
alcohol intake, obesity, poor exercise tolerance and saddle pressure
from bicycle riding.

Smoking

A literature review of eighteen studies revealed the detrimental effect
of smoking on erectile function (Dorey, 2001b). Smoking has been
found to compromise the peripheral circulation due to contraction of
the smooth muscle in the arterioles. Also, data suggest that sexual dysfunction worsens as chronic obstructive lung disease worsens (Fletcher
and Martin, 1982). Smokers were one and a half times more likely to
suffer erectile dysfunction than non-smokers. Cessation of smoking
may restore normal function (Mikhailidis et al., 1998). The review presented strong reasons for stopping smoking and highlighted the need
for a comprehensive smoking cessation programme.

Conversely, analysis from the Male Massachusetts Aging Study
(MMAS) indicated that a change in smoking status was not associated
with decreased risk for erectile dysfunction ($p > 0.03$) (Derby et al.,
2000b). However, the study was limited to only two time points and the
sample size in each category was small.

High alcohol intake

Excess intake of alcohol can lead to erectile difficulties (Fabra and
Porst, 1999; Tan and Philip, 1999), though analysis from the MMAS
indicated that a change in heavy drinking was not associated with
decreased risk for ED ($p > 0.3$) (Derby et al., 2000b).

Obesity

Data from the MMAS study showed that obesity status is associated
with erectile dysfunction ($p = 0.006$), with baseline obesity predicting
a higher risk regardless of follow-up weight loss (Derby et al., 2000b).
By the fifth and sixth decade the long-term physiological effects of obesity may be difficult to reverse (Derby et al., 2000b).

Hypertension, hypercholesterolemia and diabetes are more common
in obese patients than those who are not overweight. The survey
defined obesity in men as those with a body mass index of 27.8 kg/m^2 or
greater. Obese patients have an increased prevalence of vascular risk
factors compared with non-obese men; this imposes a risk of vasculo-
genic erectile dysfunction ($p < 0.05$) (Chung et al., 1999). Chung et al.
(1999) classified obesity as >120 per cent of ideal body weight.

Sedentary lifestyle

Analysis of the MMAS indicated that sedentary behaviour was associated with erectile dysfunction ($p = 0.01$), with the highest risk among men who remained sedentary and the lowest among those who remained active or initiated physical activity (Derby et al., 2000a). Physical activity may reduce the risk of erectile dysfunction even if initiated in midlife (Derby et al., 2000a). This may be due to a reversal of cardiovascular changes.

Saddle pressure

Perineal trauma may result from the use of a hard saddle when bicycling, horse riding or driving a tractor. Continued pressure from a hard saddle may cause paralysis of the pelvic floor muscles from pudendal nerve compression (Amarenco et al., 1987). Schwarzer et al. (2002) found that perineal pressure compressed the perineal arteries and decreased penile oxygen. They recommended a wide saddle to avoid perineal artery compression.

Lifestyle changes

The literature shows that smoking, a high consumption of alcohol, obesity, poor exercise tolerance and saddle pressure from bicycle riding are known risk factors for erectile dysfunction. Changing lifestyle in these areas may improve health and well-being and improve penile erection. Lifestyle changes can be monitored by recording the number of cigarettes smoked a day, the daily units of alcohol intake, weekly weight gain or loss, the amount of daily exercise undertaken and the miles cycled each week.

Chapter 3
Methodology of the trial

The primary purpose of this study was to determine whether pelvic floor muscle exercises and manometric biofeedback can alleviate erectile dysfunction. The secondary and lesser objective was to assess the data for possible beneficial effects of pelvic floor muscle exercises and manometric biofeedback on post-micturition dribble.

Ethical considerations

Prior to the trial, consideration was given to a range of important ethical issues as documented by the Research Governance Framework for Health and Social Care (2001). It was paramount that the participants should be able to give informed consent to participate in the trial. It was important that they understood the sampling process, the amount of involvement, the invasive nature of the digital anal examination, the use of the anal pressure probe and their rights as trial participants. Ethical considerations, therefore, included providing detailed written information about all aspects of the study, notifying their GP, gaining written informed consent, allowing men to withdraw at any time from the study, providing contacts for adverse events, finding secure storage for records and maintaining patient and partner confidentiality. Ethics approval was granted prior to the study from Taunton and Somerset NHS Trust Research and Development Executive Group, West Somerset Local Research Ethics Committee, and the University of the West of England, Bristol, Ethics Committee.

During the trial there were difficulties in recruiting a sufficient number of participants directly from the consultant urologist. Therefore, ethical approval was sought for the researcher to request referrals to the urologist from local GPs. A letter to the GPs was submitted and ethical approval was granted.

Role as clinical specialist

The researcher was a specialist continence physiotherapist, with experience in treating male continence patients and therefore well placed to combine these dual roles and undertake the trial. There were potential problems when the researcher was the clinician conducting the trial. Throughout the trial, from the initial design stage to the final analysis, the researcher was aware of the risk of bias. Steps were taken to minimise bias through the design of a randomised controlled trial, the use of validated questionnaires, objective outcome measures for measuring pelvic floor muscle strength, and the involvement of a blind assessor. Care was taken during the trial to give the intervention group and the control group the same amount of encouragement and optimism and the same number of treatment sessions, and to provide similar verbal motivation in order to avoid any bias during data collection.

Research design

As the literature review failed to identify any grade I or grade II evidence-based trials, a randomised controlled trial was designed to explore the effectiveness of pelvic floor muscle exercises for men with erectile dysfunction. The trial was designed to compare an intervention group of men with ED who received pelvic floor muscle exercises enhanced by manometric biofeedback and lifestyle changes with a control group of men with ED who were recommended lifestyle changes only. Patients were assessed by a consultant urologist, who was unaware of the group to which they were assigned. Difficulties in recruitment led to the crossover parallel arm design so that men in the control group were offered the intervention after three months.

Inclusion criteria

Men aged 20 years and over who had experienced erectile dysfunction for six months or more were included in the trial.

Exclusion criteria

Men with urological congenital abnormalities, neurological deficits and previous urological surgery (with the exception of a transurethral resection of prostate) were excluded from the trial.

Sample

The initial sample consisted of 56 men. One man was immediately excluded as he worked abroad.

Recruitment

Men were referred for treatment by a consultant urologist at a local general hospital in Taunton and GPs were invited to 'fast track' suitable patients to the urologist to encourage greater recruitment to the trial.

Setting

Men were treated by the clinician in the outpatient department of a local general hospital in Taunton. The clinician undertook the dual role of specialist continence physiotherapist and researcher.

Protocol

1. A random number system of odd or even tickets in sealed envelopes for patient selection was used to randomise patients into the intervention or the control group. Men selected and opened their sealed envelope from a box containing 150 sealed envelopes. Those who selected a ticket with an even number entered the intervention group.

2. Both groups were invited to sign the consent form and complete the International Index of Erectile Function (IIEF) (Appendix 1) and the Erectile Dysfunction-Effect on Quality of Life (ED-EQoL) (Appendix 2). All the men were requested to ask if their partner would like to sign a consent form and complete the Partner's IIEF (PIIEF) (Appendix 3). Men took the PIIEF home and were told that the partner should complete it unaided. The partner returned the PIIEF and the consent form to the clinician in a stamped addressed envelope.

3. Both groups were asked initial questions concerning the stability of relationship, the type of relationship, the number of relationships and the source of referral.

4. Both groups underwent full subjective assessment. This included questions relating to age, occupation and hobbies, the difficulty gaining and/or maintaining penile erection, premature ejaculation and duration of erectile dysfunction (Appendix 4). All subjects were asked if they had urinary and/or faecal leakage and/or post-micturition dribble. The surgical history section included questions concerning radical prostatectomy and transurethral resection of prostate, while the medical history section was designed to reveal conditions such as prostatitis, latex allergy, heart problems, blood pressure problems, serious back or neck problems, medications, diabetes and neurological problems.

5. Both groups underwent an objective assessment. This included height and weight in order to calculate the Body Mass Index

(Appendix 5). The examination was conducted in supine lying with knees bent and feet on couch to determine the ability to perform a penile retraction and scrotal lift. An assessment was made of the puborectalis muscle strength and the length of hold of the contraction in seconds by digital anal examination graded 0 (nil) to 5 (strong). An assessment of muscle strength was performed using anal manometry, with each subject positioned in supine lying as before and with a view of the computer screen for feedback. An air-filled sheathed and lubricated anal probe with a diameter of 1 cm was inserted into the anal canal to a depth of 4 cm in order to approximate to the puborectalis muscle. Subjects were instructed to tighten and lift the pelvic floor muscles as strongly as possible as if preventing the flow of urine and to hold this contraction for ten seconds (Burgio et al., 1989; Savoye et al., 2000). The clinician observed a scrotal lift and penile retraction to ascertain that the pelvic floor muscles were contracting correctly. The maximum anal pressure reading achieved from the best of three pelvic floor muscle contractions ('maximum anal pressure') and the lowest pressure obtained while attempting to maintain a ten-second hold ('anal hold pressure') were recorded in cmH_2O. A rest of ten seconds was given between each contraction.

6. Men in the intervention group were educated about the mechanics of the pelvic floor musculature and individually taught specific pelvic floor muscle exercises enhanced with manometric biofeedback for strength and endurance. The exercise programme included lifting the pelvic floor muscles 50 per cent of maximum whilst walking occasionally and a post-void 'squeeze-out' muscle contraction (Appendix 6). These treatments were given in five 30-minute periods in consecutive weeks and included advice on lifestyle changes concerning smoking, alcohol intake, general fitness, a healthy diet, weight reduction and saddle pressure (Appendix 7). Each subject in the intervention group was given a list of home exercises.

7. Men in the control group were given advice only on lifestyle changes in five 30-minute periods in consecutive weeks. No pelvic floor muscle exercises were recommended for men in this group.

8. Men in the control group were offered the opportunity to cross over into the intervention group at three months and were assessed by digital anal examination, anal manometry, ED-EQoL, IIEF and PIIEF questionnaires at baseline, three, six and nine months.

9. Men in the intervention group were assessed by digital anal examination, anal manomtery and ED-EQoL, IIEF, and PIIEF questionnaires at baseline, three and six months.

10. Men receiving intervention in both groups who experienced post-micturition dribble were given a weighed dribble-collector pad to

wear for 24 hours, with instructions to place it in a sealed bag after use. It was then weighed again.

11. A consultant urologist, who was blinded to the grouping, monitored the erectile dysfunction status and post-micturition dribble status at three and six months for subjects in the intervention group and at three, six and nine months for subjects in the control group. Subjects were asked the following standard questions: 'How is your erectile function now?' 'How is your post-micturition dribble?' 'How is your urinary leakage?' 'Do you want to continue your current treatment?' and 'How do you feel now compared to how you felt when you entered the study?' (Appendix 8).

Data analysis

In addition to the statistical advice received in the design aspects of the trial from the supervisory team, Dr Paul Ewings, statistician for the Taunton and Somerset NHS Trust Research and Development Executive Group, has offered advice with data analysis.

The researcher collected data from the subjective assessment, the IIEF, PIIEF and ED-EQoL questionnaires, and objective data from the digital anal examination and anal manometric measurements of the intervention group at baseline, at three months and six months, and of the control group at baseline, three, six and nine months. Data were coded and entered into the statistical package SPSS® for initial data analysis and comparison of the intervention and control groups.

Changes as a function of time within and between men in the intervention and control groups were assessed for erectile function using outcomes from the IIEF, PIIEF and ED-EQoL questionnaires. The distribution of data from the erectile function domain of the IIEF was found to be abnormal from a Kolmogorov-Smirnov test for normality. A non-parametric Mann-Whitney Test was performed on the erectile function domain of the IIEF for both groups at three months for evidence of variance. The data were analysed for a clinical shift of six points in the Erectile Domain of the IIEF (Goldstein, 2000). A Kolmogorov-Smirnov test of normality showed normal distribution for IIEF and PIIEF data, which were compared for evidence of correlation using Pearson's correlation coefficient. A Kolmogorov-Smirnov test of normality showed normal distribution for ED-EQoL data, so an independent samples t-test was performed for both groups at three months for evidence of variance. The ED-EQoL data were compared with the IIEF using Pearson's correlation. The erectile function domain of the IIEF was compared for evidence of correlation with the ED-EQoL using Spearman's correlation coefficient.

Changes as a function of time within and between men in the intervention and control groups were assessed for pelvic floor muscle strength using outcomes from anal manometry and digital anal examination. Anal manometric measurements failed to yield a normal distribution and were compared for evidence of variance for both groups at three months using a Mann-Whitney U independent samples test. Ordinal data from digital anal measurements were compared for evidence of variance for both groups at three months using a non-parametric paired Wilcoxon test. The relationship between pelvic floor muscle strength and severity of erectile dysfunction was analysed. Anal manometric measurements were compared with the erectile function domain of the IIEF for evidence of correlation using Spearman's correlation coefficient for two-tailed bivariate correlation. Digital anal measurements were compared with the erectile function domain of the IIEF for evidence of correlation using non-parametric bivariate two-tailed Spearman's correlation coefficient. Anal manometric measurements were compared with digital anal measurements for evidence of correlation using non-parametric bivariate two-tailed Spearman's correlation coefficient.

Analysis of covariance was performed to confirm or challenge the between group difference at three months controlling for the Erectile Function at baseline and the maximum anal pressure at baseline.

Separate analysis was performed on the control group who received intervention after three months. A Wilcoxon paired samples test was performed on the Erectile Function domain of the IIEF for evidence of variance between baseline, at three, six and nine months for the control group. A paired samples t-test was performed on data from the ED-EQoL.

Linear regression analysis using natural logged data of the dependent variable was used to identify predictors among sub-groups of men with erectile dysfunction, for smoking, alcohol intake, anti-hypertensive medication, body mass index, duration of erectile dysfunction and age.

Outcome measures for post-micturition dribble were analysed from the categories used in the blind assessment of 'worse', 'same', 'less leakage', 'less leakage, less often' and 'cured'. The relationship between pelvic floor muscle strength and presence of post-micturition dribble was assessed using non-parametric bivariate two-tailed Spearman's correlation coefficient. Anal manometric measurements were compared with post-micturition status for evidence of correlation using two-tailed Spearman's correlation coefficient. Digital anal measurements were compared with post-micturition status at baseline for evidence of correlation using Spearman's correlation coefficient.

Chapter 4
Methodology: developmental issues

Before the trial commenced a number of issues needed to be addressed. These included a reliability analysis of the anal pressure probe, the development of a questionnaire for partners and the selection of the most appropriate outcome measures.

Reliability analysis of the anal pressure probe

Introduction

In order to analyse the reliability of the anal pressure measurements, a within-day and day-to-day reliability study was undertaken. Anal manometry with an air-filled pressure probe has previously been used to monitor the strength of pelvic floor muscles for men with urinary incontinence (Burgio et al., 1989), for men before and after radical prostatectomy (Sueppel et al., 2001) and for faecal incontinence (Norton et al., 2000). No reliability studies have been conducted on this technique as a method of measuring pelvic floor muscle strength.

Objective

A test–retest design was used to assess within-day and day-to-day reliability of anal manometric measurements taken with the ECL F2 Elite System (Genesis Medical Ltd, London), in a group of out-patients with self-reported erectile dysfunction.

Methods

Subjects

Twenty-six men from the erectile dysfunction trial read the information sheet gave informed consent to take part in this reliability study and completed the consent form. A consecutive sample of ten men from

the intervention group was selected for assessment of within-day reliability of anal manometric measurements. A further cohort of sixteen
men was selected from the control group for day-to-day reliability
analysis. The description of subjects is shown in Table 4.1.

Table 4.1: Description of subjects in reliability studies

	Within-Day Reliability	Day-to-Day Reliability
Number of subjects	10	16
Mean age	54 years	55 years
Age range	33–67 years	43–69 years
Mean height	1.79 metres	1.79 metres
Height range	1.65–1.88 metres	1.75–1.88 metres
Mean body mass index	27.83	29.50
Body mass index range	22–35	2–42

Ethical permission was obtained from the West Somerset Local
Research Ethics Committee, the Taunton and Somerset NHS Trust
Research and Development Executive Group and the University of the
West of England, Bristol, Ethics Committee.

Calibration of instrument

Prior to the reliability study, incremental measurements of pressure
taken by manually squeezing the anal pressure probe connected to the
ECL F2 Elite System were compared with a standard manometer, which
had previously been calibrated to International Standards. Pressure
readings were compared in laboratory conditions across the range
15 cmH$_2$O–210 cmH$_2$O, which represented the range of measurements
recorded in everyday clinical use of the probe.

Assessment of reliability

To assess within-day reliability, measurements were taken from men
receiving pelvic floor muscle exercises as part of the current trial. Each
subject was positioned in supine lying with two pillows under his head,
with knees bent and feet on the couch and a view of the computer
screen for feedback (Dorey, 2001c). The screen displayed no scale or
goal line. The air-filled, sheathed and lubricated anal probe was inserted into the anal canal as far as the external position marker in order to
approximate to the puborectalis muscle (Dorey, 2001c) (Figure 4.1).
   Subjects were instructed to tighten and lift the pelvic floor muscles
as strongly as possible and hold this contraction for ten seconds (Burgio

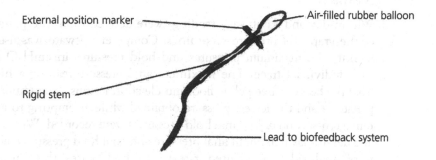

External position marker

Air-filled rubber balloon

Rigid stem

Lead to biofeedback system

Figure 4.1: Anal pressure probe

et al., 1989; Savoye et al., 2000) (Figure 4.2). Three attempts were made at this test sequence with ten seconds' rest between attempts. The clinician observed a scrotal lift and penile retraction to ascertain that the pelvic floor muscles were contracting. Following the three trials, the anal probe was removed and the patient allowed to relax. The entire procedure was repeated after an interval of five minutes with the subject blind to any previous readings or graphic traces.

To assess day-to-day reliability the test procedure was repeated at the same time of day (± 2 hours) because of possible diurnal fluctuations in anal pressure following a three-month interval. These subjects received no pelvic floor muscle training during this period.

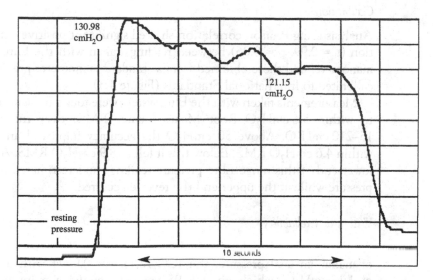

130.98 cmH$_2$O

121.15 cmH$_2$O

resting pressure

10 seconds

Figure 4.2: Computer trace showing anal pressure during one testing cycle

Analysis

Within-day and day-to-day readings were derived from interpretation of the graphs of pressure recordings. Computer software was used to identify the maximum pressures and hold pressures in cmH_2O from each individual trace. The maximum anal pressure reading achieved from the best of three pelvic floor muscle contractions ('maximum anal pressure') and the lowest pressure obtained while attempting to maintain a ten-second hold ('anal hold pressure') were recorded. Within-day and day-to-day maximum anal pressure and anal hold pressure readings were analysed using paired t-tests. In both cases the Intraclass Correlation Coefficient (ICC) (2,1) and Standard Error of Measurement (SEM) were also calculated.

$$ICC\ (2,1) = \cfrac{BMS - RMS}{\cfrac{BMS + (k-1)\ RMS + k(TMS - RMS)}{N}}$$

Where: BMS = Between Subjects Mean Squares
RMS = Residual Mean Square
TMS = Treatments Mean Square
k   = number of observers
N   = subjects being examined

Results

Calibration

Analysis using Pearson correlation showed significant positive correlation ($r = 0.99$, $p = 0.06$) between readings taken with the Elite anal manometer and those obtained from a standard manometer previously calibrated to International Standards (Figure 4.3).

Measurements taken with the Elite system were found to be accurate to within 5.6 cmH_2O Root Mean Square (RMS) over the range 15–210 cmH_2O. Above 50 cmH_2O the accuracy improved and was within 4.6 cmH_2O RMS. Below this it fell to 8.9 cmH_2O RMS. At the lower end of this range Elite pressure readings underestimated actual pressure while at the upper end the reverse occurred.

Within-day reliability

Results are summarised in Table 4.2 and Figure 4.4. For measurements of maximum anal pressure, the ICC (2,1) was 0.9994 with a SEM of 1.17 cmH_2O, which gives a 95 per cent confidence interval of

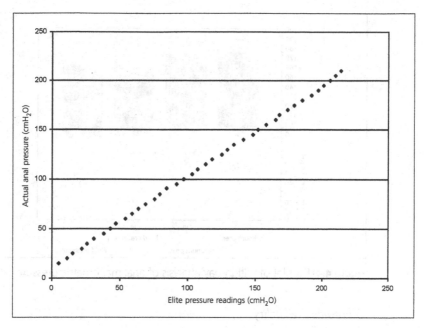

Figure 4.3: Accuracy of the Elite anal manometer readings (cmH$_2$O) (r = 0.99)

Table 4.2: Table of results

Pressure CmH$_2$O	Within-Day Measurements (n = 10)				Day-to-Day Measurements (n = 16)			
	Maximum Anal Pressure		Anal Hold Pressure		Maximum Anal Pressure		Anal Hold Pressure	
Measurement	M1	M2	M1	M2	M1	M3	M1	M3
Mean	127.0	127.3	117.6	118.1	76.4	76.2	70.3	70.5
SD	48.0	47.9	45.3	45.5	24.7	23.1	23.4	22.4
Range	40–188	41–190	36–178	37–178	13–112	15–101	11–112	12–99
t-test p	0.58		0.30		0.94		0.93	
ICC (2,1)	0.9994		0.9995		0.9151		0.9258	
SEM	1.17		3.21		6.76		6.06	
95% CI	127.15 ± 2.34		117.85 ± 6.42		76.3 ± 13.52		70.4 ± 12.12	

± 2.34 cmH$_2$O (Denagar and Ball, 1993). For measurements of anal hold pressure the ICC (2,1) was 0.9995 with a SEM of 3.21 cmH$_2$O and 95 per cent confidence intervals of ± 6.42 cmH$_2$O. There were no significant differences between repeated measurements of maximum anal pressure (p = 0.58) or anal hold pressure (p = 0.30).

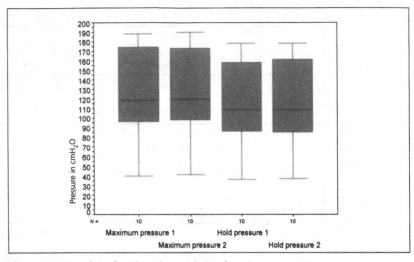

Figure 4.4: Boxplot of within-day analysis of anal manometric pressure

Day-to-day reliability

Results are summarised in Table 4.2 and Figure 4.5. For measurements of maximum anal pressure, the ICC (2,1) was calculated to be 0.9151 with a SEM of 6.76 cmH$_2$O and 95 per cent confidence intervals of ± 13.52 cmH$_2$O. The equivalent results for anal hold pressures were ICC (2,1) 0.9258, SEM 6.06 cmH$_2$O and 95 per cent confidence intervals ± 12.12 cmH$_2$O. There were no significant differences between repeated measurements of maximum anal pressure (p = 0.94) or anal hold pressure (p = 0.93).

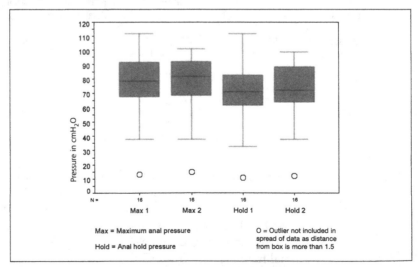

Figure 4.5: Boxplot of day-to-day analysis of anal manometric pressure

Discussion

This study investigated the within-day and day-to-day reproducibility of the anal pressure probe ECL F2 Elite System (Genesis Medical Ltd, London). Anal pressure measurements using this equipment were found to demonstrate good accuracy, particularly above 50 cmH$_2$O, which represented the lower limit of clinical measurements of pressure in 88 per cent of subjects. Below 50 cmH$_2$O accuracy declined to 8.9 cmH$_2$O RMS. Overall, these levels of accuracy, which were within 10 cmH$_2$O, can be considered to be clinically acceptable.

Differences may also be attributable to variations in pelvic floor muscle strength, age, body mass index (BMI) and different physiques and fitness of the subjects. The anal pressure measurements in this sample of men with erectile dysfunction varied considerably from 11 cmH$_2$O to 190 cmH$_2$O. Pressures recorded were lower for day-to-day analysis (11–112 cmH$_2$O, mean 76.4 cmH$_2$O), where subjects were selected from the control group of the current trial, than for within-day analysis (40–190 cmH$_2$O, mean 127.0 cmH$_2$O), where subjects were from the intervention group of this trial and therefore recipients of pelvic floor muscle training.

In this study, the best of three attempts at maximum pelvic floor muscle contraction was used as a measure of optimal performance. However, other studies have used different approaches. Fynes et al. (1999), for example, recorded the mean of three readings. They took anal measurements in women; therefore direct comparison with the results of men in this study was not possible. In the current study, anal hold pressure was recorded in addition to maximum pressure to give an indication of the strength of the pelvic floor muscle contraction after a ten-second delay. This time period has been used in clinical studies of pelvic floor muscle re-education (Moore et al., 1999; Van Kampen et al., 2000). However, these studies, and a study incorporating a shorter hold of five seconds (Wyndaele and Van Eetvelde, 1996), do not report hold pressures.

Wyndaele and Van Eetvelde (1996) found that digital anal examination of both the external anal sphincter and the puborectalis muscle was reliable after intervals of ten seconds, two hours and four hours. However, direct comparisons with this study are not meaningful as their sample consisted of healthy young men with a mean age of 24.5 years, unlike the wider age group of men with erectile dysfunction used in this study.

Results indicated good within-day reliability of measurements taken with the anal probe. Day-to-day reliability incorporated additional sources of variation such as subject position and reinsertion of the anal probe. However day-to-day reliability was good for both maximum anal pressure and anal hold pressure and comparable with within-day reliability. Intraclass Correlation Coefficients indicate the retest variability relative to the differences between subjects. They are a proportional index and high variability between subjects as seen in this study therefore tends to return a high ICC (Keating and Matyas, 1998). The high ICCs observed suggested that anal pressure measurements were very useful for discriminating between individual subjects in a group of patients under study (Bland and Altman, 1996). The high reliability may also be due to a number of methodological factors. There was only one experienced clinician taking measurements. Reliability may be reduced by multiple raters, particularly if they are inexperienced. In this study the large subject age range (33–69 years) may have contributed to the range of anal pressures found. Another factor that may have contributed to the good reliability of results is that maximum anal pressure, based on the best of three contractions, is more likely to return a reliable result than single pressure measurements. The standard error of measurement can be used to calculate 95 per cent confidence limits about a given measurement. As expected, these are lower for within-day compared to day-to-day measures and may reflect additional sources of variation in the latter.

Potential sources of variation of anal pressure probe measurements, such as subject position, rectal contents and atmospheric pressure, do not appear to have significantly compromised the reliability of results. These factors were taken into account in the study design as men were tested in the same position, seen at the same time of day, were given standardised instructions, and the anal probe was inserted to the same depth each time. The sample was also apparently not significantly affected by factors that might have influenced patient effort, such as enthusiasm, discomfort, mood and past experience of anal examination.

The findings in this trial suggested reliable measurements of anal pressure were obtainable on both a day-to-day and within-day basis. It would be interesting to compare anal manometry with anal EMG and digital anal examination to investigate a possible association. These three methods of assessment have been shown to be significantly correlated when carried out vaginally (Haslam, 1999).

The findings of this study suggested that clinically reliable measurements of anal pressure were obtainable in men with erectile dysfunction. Further studies are needed to assess the inter-rater reliability of anal pressure measurements since more than one clinician may be involved in the assessment of muscle strength over time. The findings of reliability studies related only to the group under study. Assessment of reliability in more heterogeneous cohorts of men, including healthy men, and those with distinct pathology linked to erectile or urological dysfunction, would be useful in the further assessment of the clinical utility of this procedure.

The validity of anal pressure measurements in the assessment of pelvic floor muscle strength also needs to be determined, for example, by comparison of the results of anal manometry with anal EMG.

Conclusion

Reliable clinical measurements of anal pressure were obtainable in a group of men with erectile difficulties. Anal manometry may be a useful clinical measurement in the assessment of men with erectile and continence problems.

Development of the Partner's International Index of Erectile Function

The Partner's International Index of Erectile Function (PIIEF) was compiled by the author to mirror the questions contained in the IIEF in order to involve the partner and obtain a second opinion on the level of erectile dysfunction (Appendix 3). It was developed to confirm the accuracy of male reporting. It has not been validated. The PIIEF contained fifteen questions which were ranked 0 (No sexual activity), 1 (Almost never or never), 2 (A few times), 3 (Sometimes), 4 (Most times) and 5 (Almost always or always), giving a maximum potential total of 75 points.

In future studies a partner's questionnaire could monitor the partner's perception of the problem rather than mirror the questions in the IIEF. Partners may have different needs. They may place more value on touch, closeness and other forms of sexual activity, which do not include vaginal penetration. They may consider the relationship to be more important than the desire for sexual intercourse. Partners may be male with different sexual needs. Validation of such a questionnaire should include input from partners of different preferences, ages, cultures and religions.

Selection of outcome measures for the current trial

The literature review of outcome measures used to monitor treatment efficacy for men with erectile dysfunction revealed a number of subjective and objective outcome measures. Selection of the appropriate measurement tool was challenging, since no measure was able to express fully the outcome of an intervention (Mattiasson et al., 1998). The following outcome measures were selected for this trial.

International Index of Erectile Function

The International Index of Erectile Function (IIEF) was chosen as the main outcome measure as it was found to provide a psychometrically sound, reliable, validated assessment of erectile function (Rosen et al., 1997) (Appendix 1). The Erectile Function domain of the IIEF consisted of questions 1, 2, 3, 4, 5 and 15, which were ranked 0 (No sexual activity), 1 (Almost never or never), 2 (A few times), 3 (Sometimes), 4 (Most times), 5 (Almost always or always) giving a possible maximum score of 30 for good erectile function. Goldstein (2000) classified erectile dysfunction according to the score in Erectile Function domain as 0–6 points severe dysfunction, 7–12 points moderate–severe, 13–18 points moderate, 19–24 points mild and 25–30 points normal function (Table 2.5). An increase of six or more points in the erectile function domain was considered to signify a clinical improvement (Goldstein, 2000).

Partner's International Index of Erectile Function

The Partner's International Index of Erectile Function was compiled by the author to mirror the questions contained in the IIEF in order to involve the partner and verify the subject's response (Appendix 3). It has not yet been validated.

Erectile Dysfunction – Effect on Quality of Life

The Erectile Dysfunction Effect on Quality of Life (ED-EQoL), the only validated ED-specific quality of life questionnaire, was chosen to complement the IIEF and provide a quality of life perspective (MacDonagh et al., 2002). There were fifteen questions (Appendix 2). Each question had five possible responses scored 0–4 and the fifteen scores were summed to give a total score of 0 (good QoL) to 60 (poor QoL).

Anal manometry

Anal manometry was chosen for the trial as a reliable measure of assessing the squeeze pressure in cmH_2O of the puborectalis muscle reinforced by the pelvic floor musculature (Dorey and Swinkels, 2002). The maximum anal pressure reading achieved from the best of three pelvic floor muscle contractions ('maximum anal pressure') and the lowest pressure obtained while attempting to maintain a ten-second hold ('anal hold pressure') could be recorded in cmH_2O.

Digital anal examination

Digital anal examination was chosen as a valid and reliable method outcome measure of assessing puborectalis muscle strength (Wyndaele and Van Eetvelde, 1996). Muscles could be graded 0–5 for muscle strength (see Table 2.6) and the length of contraction in seconds monitored.

Blind assessment

There is a potential for bias when the clinician is also the researcher undertaking the trial. Such influences are common and are known as 'experimenter bias effects'. These influences may be unintentional and unconscious, particularly where data involve subjective reporting (Hicks, 1995). To allay this type of bias, one solution is to operate a single 'blind' procedure where the assessor is unaware of the hypothesis being tested. In this trial, the consultant urologist assessed subjects using standard questions without knowledge of the subject's grouping, at three and six months for the intervention group and three, six and nine months for the control group (Appendix 8).

Chapter 5
Results

Introduction

First, results are reported from the important randomised controlled component of the trial, which compared the effect of three months' intervention (pelvic floor muscle exercises, manometric biofeedback and advice on lifestyle changes) with the effect of three months' advice on lifestyle changes recommended to the control group. Results are also given of the effect of a further three months of home exercises performed by subjects in the intervention group.

Second, results are reported from the parallel arm of the trial, where the control group crossed over at the three-month assessment and received three months' intervention followed by a further three months of home exercises. The control group who crossed over into the parallel arm are termed the control group throughout.

The flow of subjects through this randomised controlled trial with a cross-over parallel arm is shown in an algorithm (Figure 5.1).

Description of subjects

Fifty-six subjects were recruited into the trial; one subject dropped out before randomisation. Twenty-eight subjects were randomised into the intervention group and twenty-seven into the control group. At the three-month assessment, the control group crossed over to receive the intervention. For both groups the intervention was followed by three months of home exercises (Figure 5.1). The subjects were compared for between-group differences in age, body mass index and duration of erectile dysfunction at baseline (Table 5.1). The distribution of the age of the subjects displayed on a histogram also showed a normal distribution curve. A Kolmogorov-Smirnov test for normality showed $p = 0.090$ significance, which enabled statistical analysis by parametric

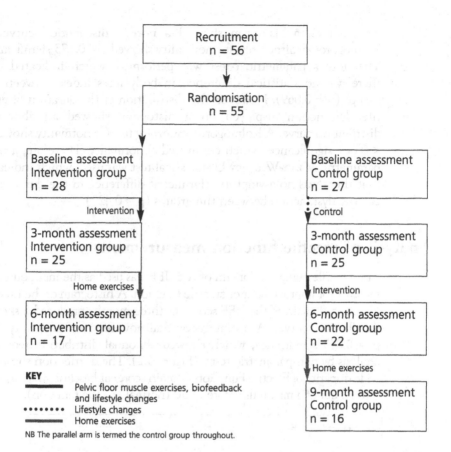

Figure 5.1: Algorithm of randomised controlled trial with cross-over parallel arm

tests. Therefore, a t-test was performed, which indicated that there was no statistical significant difference in age between the groups (p = 0.082). The distribution of the body mass index of the subjects

Table 5.1: Description of subjects at baseline

Description	Intervention Group	Control Group	Test	Sig.p
Number of subjects	28	27	–	–
Mean age (SD)	53.9 years (13.0)	59.2 years (8.62)	t-test	0.082
Median age	57.5 years	61.0 years	–	–
Age range	22–78 years	41–72 years	–	–
Mean body mass index (SD)	26.9 (4.1)	28.8 (3.41)	t-test	0.069
Body mass index range	21–42	22–38	–	–
Mean months with ED	76.6	68.1	U test	0.427
Months with ED range	6–360	6–360	–	–

displayed on a histogram showed a normal distribution curve. A Kolmogorov-Smirnov test for normality showed p = 0.173 significance. Therefore a parametric t-test was performed, which indicated that there was no statistical difference in body mass index between the groups (p = 0.069). However, the distribution of the duration of erectile dysfunction displayed on a histogram showed an abnormal distribution curve. A Kolmogorov-Smirnov test for normality showed p < 0.001 significance, which confirmed abnormality. Therefore, a non-parametric Mann-Whitney U statistical test was used, which indicated that there was no asymptotic significant difference in the duration of erectile dysfunction between the groups (p = 0.427).

Analysis of erectile function measurements

The Erectile Function domain of the IIEF was used as the main outcome measure for improvement of erectile function. A histogram of the Erectile Function domain of the IIEF scores at three months produced a skewed distribution curve. A Kolmogorov-Smirnov test for normality had p = 0.003 significance, which showed abnormal distribution requiring analysis by non-parametric tests. (Figure 5.2). The distribution showed a wide disparity of Erectile Function domain scores at baseline ranging from 0 to 28 out of a maximum score of 30 (normal erectile function).

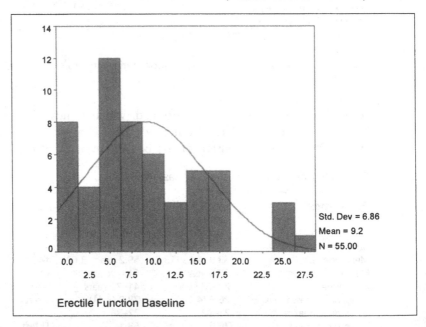

Figure 5.2: Histogram showing baseline distribution of Erectile Function domain of IIEF scores

The distribution curves for the IIEF and ED-EQoL at baseline also produced normal distribution curves. A Kolmogorov-Smirnov test for normality showed significances of P = 0.200 and p = 0.200 respectively, which allowed parametric approaches.

The mean IIEF individual scores (0–5) for each question showed an improvement following intervention and home exercises for both groups. Also the mean total scores of the Erectile Function domain of the IIEF (0–30) showed a marked improvement following intervention and home exercises in both groups (the bottom line in Table 5.2).

In this mixed cross-over parallel arm trial, the important randomised controlled part of the trial compared the intervention group with the

Table 5.2: Mean International Index of Erectile Function scores for both groups at three-monthly intervals

Mean IIEF scores	Intervention (n = 28)			Control (n = 27)			
Months from baseline	0	3	6	0	3	6	9
Sample number	28	25	17	27	25	22	16
1 Frequency of erection	1.9	3.2	3.8	1.7	1.5	3.3	3.5
2 Frequency of hard erections	1.8	3.2	3.7	1.3	1.4	3.1	3.1
3 Ability to penetrate	1.8	3.0	3.4	1.3	1.4	3.2	3.3
4 Rigidity after penetration	1.6	2.7	3.0	1.0	1.2	3.1	2.8
5 Ability to complete intercourse	1.7	2.6	3.1	1.3	1.0	2.9	2.8
6 Number of intercourse attempts	1.6	2.0	2.1	1.5	1.4	2.0	2.3
7 Intercourse satisfaction	1.8	3.0	3.0	1.3	1.6	2.8	3.1
8 Intercourse enjoyment	1.9	2.7	2.8	1.7	1.6	2.9	3.1
9 Frequency of ejaculation	2.2	3.4	3.6	1.9	2.0	3.2	3.0
10 Frequency of orgasm	1.6	3.3	3.6	2.3	2.0	3.6	3.0
11 Frequency of sexual desire	1.2	3.3	3.2	1.7	3.1	3.7	3.8
12 Level of sexual desire	1.4	2.9	3.1	1.7	2.8	3.4	3.4
13 Sex life satisfaction	1.1	2.9	3.2	1.5	1.9	3.0	3.2
14 Relationship satisfaction	1.5	3.2	3.4	2.1	2.2	3.1	3.1
15 Erection confidence	1.7	2.6	3.2	1.9	1.7	2.7	3.1
Mean IIEF out of 75	30.5	42.7	48.0	26.0	27.0	46.0	46.6
Mean Erectile Function domain (Questions 1, 2, 3, 4, 5 and 15) out of 30	10.5	17.2	20.1	7.8	8.4	18.3	18.5

KEY
 Pelvic floor muscle exercises, biofeedback and lifestyle changes
•••••••• Lifestyle changes ━━━━━━ Home exercises
NB The parallel arm is termed the control group throughout.

Erectile Function domain	=	Questions 1, 2, 3, 4, 5 and 15
Intercourse satisfaction	=	Questions 6, 7 and 8
Orgasmic function	=	Questions 9 and 10
Sexual desire	=	Questions 11 and 12
Overall satisfaction	=	Questions 13 and 14

control group at the three-month assessment. A scattergram showed the differences in erectile function between the intervention group and the control group at three months compared to baseline (Figure 5.3). This shows clearly that nine subjects (triangles) in the intervention group attained a score of 25 (normal erectile function) or over on the Erectile Function domain of the IIEF at three months (on the y axis). Closer inspection shows that six of these subjects scored low (on the x axis) at baseline, indicating that subjects with a wide disparity of scores have shown improvement in erectile function.

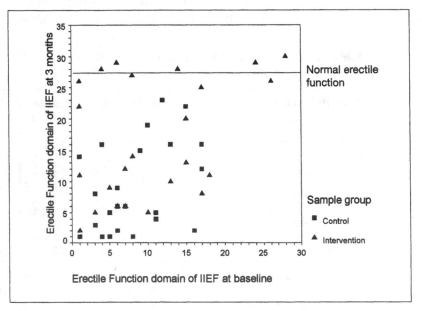

Figure 5.3: Scattergram of comparison of the Erectile Function domain of IIEF scores at baseline and three months for both groups

The intervention group showed a significant improvement (p = 0.001) in the Erectile Function domain of the IIEF compared to the control group after three months from a Mann-Whitney U test (Table 5.3). It should be noted that in the intervention group 28 subjects at baseline were compared to 25 subjects at three months as three subjects withdrew from the trial. There was also a clinical improvement of 6.74 points in the intervention group after three months compared to baseline. An increase of six points in the Erectile Function domain of the IIEF constituted a clinical improvement in which subjects moved up a category from, for example, 'Sometimes' to 'Most times' or from 'Most times' to 'Almost always'.

The control group showed only a slight improvement (0.55 points) during this period.

The results of the randomised part of the trial are displayed graphically in a boxplot (Figure 5.4). The boxes represent 50 per cent of the data and include a line marking the median. The upper and lower tails (whiskers) represent the spread of all the data. At baseline there is a larger range of Erectile Function domain scores in the intervention group than in the control group. Despite the large spread of data, the median is low, with 50 per cent of the data lying below the median line. At three months in the intervention group, there is a wide range of scores (2–30), demonstrating that some men still have a low score but some have attained high scores. However in the control group, at three months, although some men have improved the median remained the same.

Table 5.3: Results of Mann-Whitney independent samples test on Erectile Function domain on IIEF at three months for both groups

Sample	Group	Number of Men	Mean EF Domain	Range	Asymp. Sig. (2-tailed)
EF domain of IIEF at baseline	Intervention	28	10.50	1–28	0.336
	Control	27	7.81	1–17	
EF domain of IIEF at 3 months	Intervention	25	17.24	2–30	0.001*
	Control	25	8.36	1–21	

* Denotes significant difference.

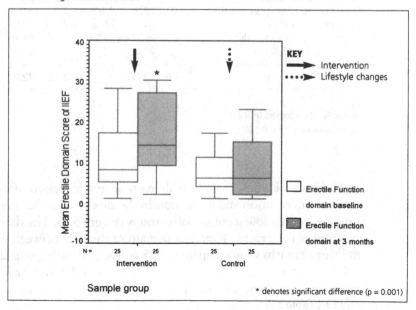

Figure 5.4: Boxplot of mean Erectile Function domain of IIEF of both groups at baseline and three months

At three months, three subjects had withdrawn from the intervention group and two had withdrawn from the control group. In the intervention group, there was a significant difference between the baseline and three-month mean scores of the Erectile Function domain of the IIEF (p = 0.008), but not for the control group (p = 0.658) when using a Wilcoxon Signed Ranks Test in 25 subjects (Table 5.4).

Table 5.4: Comparison of mean IIEF scores at baseline and three months for both groups using paired Wilcoxon Signed Ranks Test

Mean IIEF scores Months from Baseline Group	Control (n = 25)			Intervention (n = 25)		
	Baseline	3 months	p value	Baseline	3 months	p value
1 Frequency of erection	1.6	1.5	0.778	2.0	3.2	0.006*
2 Frequency of hard erections	1.2	1.4	1.000	1.9	3.2	0.004*
3 Ability to penetrate	1.2	1.4	0.868	1.9	3.0	0.011*
4 Rigidity after penetration	1.0	1.2	0.923	1.8	2.7	0.028*
5 Ability to complete intercourse	1.3	1.0	0.909	1.8	2.6	0.042*
6 Number of intercourse attempts	1.5	1.4	0.860	1.7	2.0	0.307
7 Intercourse satisfaction	1.3	1.6	0.914	1.8	3.0	0.006*
8 Intercourse enjoyment	1.8	1.6	0.987	2.0	2.7	0.085
9 Frequency of ejaculation	2.0	2.0	0.705	2.3	3.4	0.035*
10 Frequency of orgasm	1.9	2.0	0.726	2.4	3.3	0.072
11 Frequency of sexual desire	3.2	3.1	0.838	2.9	3.3	0.140
12 Level of sexual desire	2.8	2.8	0.929	2.9	2.9	1.00
13 Sex life satisfaction	1.8	1.9	1.000	2.2	2.9	0.059
14 Sexual relationship satisfaction	2.0	2.2	1.000	2.3	3.2	0.012*
15 Erection confidence	1.4	1.7	0.782	1.8	2.6	0.011*
Erectile function questions 1, 2, 3, 4, 5 and 15	7.7	8.4	0.658	11.2	17.2	0.008*
Total IIEF	25.9	27.0		31.8	42.7	

Key
Erectile Function domain of the IIEF
*Significance below p = 0.05

The mean Erectile Function domain scores increased after three months' intervention and three months' home exercises, but some men remained with a low score in both groups (Figure 5.5). The differences in scores of the Erectile Function domain of the IIEF between baseline and three months were compared in 25 subjects in each group using an independent samples t-test after applying natural logarithms to the dependent variables. The difference was found to be significant (p = 0.011) (Table 5.5).

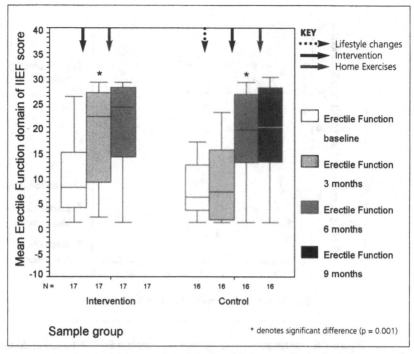

Figure 5.5: Mean Erectile Function domain of IIEF scores for both groups at each assessment

Table 5.5: Comparison of Erectile Function domain score differences between baseline and three months for intervention and control groups

Sample Group	Number of Men	Mean	Sig. EF Domain (2-tailed)
Intervention	25	6.08	0.011*
Control	25	0.76	

* Denotes significant difference.

The change in the Erectile Function domain of the IIEF of subjects in the intervention group following pelvic floor muscle exercises at three months and after home exercises at six months is portrayed in a scattergram (Figure 5.6).

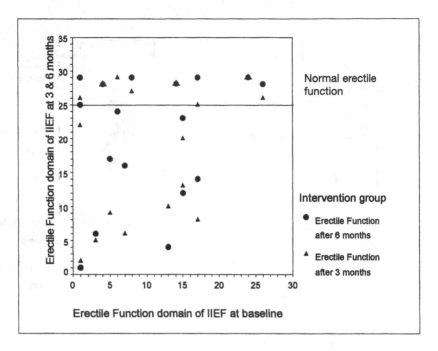

Figure 5.6: Scattergram of comparison of baseline Erectile Function domain of IIEF scores with three and six months for intervention

This scattergram showed that at baseline (on the *x* axis) subjects presented with a range of Erectile Function domain scores. Despite some of the low baseline scores, eight subjects (circles) attained a score of 25 (normal erectile function) or over after intervention and home exercises (on the *y* axis), indicating that pelvic floor muscle exercises improved erectile function in some subjects despite the severity of erectile dysfunction at baseline.

The differences in natural logged Erectile Function domain scores in the intervention group between each of the assessments were analysed separately using a paired t-test. The mean Erectile Function domain score improvement from baseline was 8 points at three months and 9.88 points at six months for the intervention group in the 17 subjects who completed the six-month assessment. The control group showed a mean difference of 0.82 points only from baseline to three months. After intervention, the control group showed a mean difference from baseline of 10.73 points at six months ($p < 0.001$) and 10.94 at nine months after home exercises ($p < 0.001$) for the sixteen subjects who completed the nine-month assessment (Table 5.6).

Table 5.6: Comparison of Erectile Function domain score differences between each assessment for both groups

Paired Differences	EF Domain Total Score Difference	Group	N	Mean Score Difference	Mean Paired Difference	Sig. (2-tailed)
Baseline to 3 months	136	Intervention	17	8.00	−6.29	0.053
3 months to 6 months	29	Intervention	17	1.71		
Baseline to 3 months	136	Intervention	17	8.00	1.88	0.122
Baseline to 6 months	168	Intervention	17	9.88		
Baseline to 3 months	18	Control	22	0.82	9.27	0.004*
3 months to 6 months	240	Control	22	10.09		
Baseline to 3 months	18	Control	22	0.82	9.91	< 0.001*
Baseline to 6 months	236	Control	22	10.73		
Baseline to 3 months	17	Control	16	1.06	9.88	< 0.001*
Baseline to 9 months	175	Control	16	10.94		

* Denotes significant difference.

When the control group crossed over to receive intervention, they continued to be referred to as the control group to avoid being confused with the intervention group. The control group was analysed separately for the effect of lifestyle changes at three months, the effect of pelvic floor muscle exercises at six months and the effect of home exercises at nine months. A scattergram showed the differences in erectile function of the control group at three, six and nine months compared to baseline (x axis) (Figure 5.7).

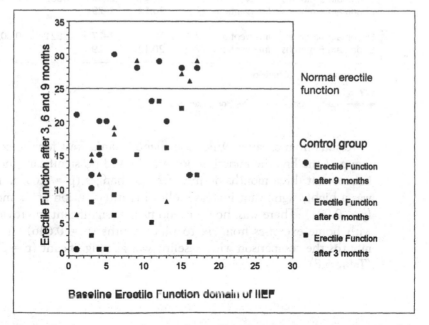

Figure 5.7: Scattergram of comparison of baseline Erectile Function domain of IIEF scores with three, six and nine months for control group

The scattergram showed that all subjects in the control group presented with a low baseline Erectile Function domain score of 17 or under (on the *x* axis), yet following intervention and home exercises, five subjects attained a score of 25 or over. The control group were analysed using a paired t-test, which showed a significant Erectile Function domain score difference between baseline and three months, and three months and six months (p = 0.004), and between baseline and three months, and baseline and nine months (p < 0.001) (Table 5.6). Statistical analysis using a paired Wilcoxon Signed Ranks Test indicated that the intervention group also had a significant improvement (p = 0.005) in the Erectile Function domain of the IIEF at six months when compared to baseline (Table 5.7). However, the improvement during home exercises from three to six months was not significant (p = 0.108).

Table 5.7: Results of paired Wilcoxon Signed Ranks Test on Erectile Function domain of IIEF at three and six months for intervention group

Paired Sample	Group	Number of Men	Mean EF Domain	Range	ρ	Sig. (2-tailed)
▼ EF domain baseline	Intervention	25	11.16	1–27	–2.635	0.008*
EF domain 3 months	Intervention	25	17.24	2–30		
↓ EF domain 3 months	Intervention	17	18.41	2–30	–1.606	0.108
▼ EF domain 6 months	Intervention	17	20.12	1–29		
▼ EF domain baseline	Intervention	17	10.41	1–27	–2.821	0.005*
↓ EF domain 6 months	Intervention	17	20.12	1–29		

* Denotes significant difference.

KEY
⟶ Intervention   ⟶ Home Exercises

Results from a paired Wilcoxon Signed Ranks Test for the control group of the Erectile Function domain showed no significant increase in scores at three months during lifestyle changes (p = 0.658). There was a highly significant increase following intervention at six months (p < 0.001). There was, however, no further significant improvement with home exercises from six to nine months (p = 0.646). At nine months the comparison with baseline was also significant (p = 0.001) (Table 5.8).

Table 5.8: Results of paired Wilcoxon Signed Ranks Test on Erectile Function domain of IIEF at three, six and nine months for control group

Paired Sample	Group	Number of Men	Mean EF Domain	Range	Z	Sig. (2-tailed)
EF domain baseline	Control	25	7.68	1–17	–0.443	0.658
EF domain 3 months	Control	25	8.36	1–21		
EF domain 3 months	Control	22	8.18	1–21	–3.606	<0.001**
EF domain 6 months	Control	22	18.27	1–29		
EF domain baseline	Control	22	7.45	1–17	–2.821	< 0.005**
EF domain 6 months	Control	22	18.27	1–29		
EF domain 6 months	Control	16	18.50	1–29	–0.460	0.646
EF domain 9 months	Control	16	18.50	1–29		
EF domain baseline	Control	16	7.87	1–17	–3.354	0.001**
EF domain 9 months	Control	16	18.50	1–29		

** Denotes significant difference.

KEY

••••▶ Lifestyle changes ⟶ Intervention ⟹ Home Exercises

At baseline, the Erectile Function domain of the IIEF was not correlated with age (rho = –0.257, p = 0.058), duration of erectile dysfunction (rho = –0.124, p = 0.367), smoking (rho = –0.043, p = 0.756), anti-hypertensive medication (rho = –0.045, p = 0.746), or body mass index (rho = 0.129, p = 0.350) when data from all subjects was analysed using Spearman's ρ correlation.

The severity of erectile dysfunction at each assessment, analysed using Spearman's correlation, failed to correlate with the Erectile Function domain at baseline for the intervention group but correlated in the control group.

The PIIEF was completed by 47 (85.5 per cent) partners at baseline. A Kolmogorov-Smirnov normality test on the distribution of the PIIEF at baseline allowed analysis using Pearson correlation. There was good correlation between the mean IIEF scores with the mean PIIEF scores for all assessments in both groups (Table 5.9). The nearer the correlation coefficient is to 1 (perfect correlation), the closer the correlation.

Table 5.9: Correlation of the mean scores of the IIEF with the PIIEF

Groups Compared	Number of Men	Pearson Correlation
Intervention IIEF baseline	28	0.956**
Intervention PIIEF baseline	23	
Intervention IIEF 3 months	25	0.715**
Intervention PIIEF 3 months	17	
Intervention IIEF 6 months	17	0.915**
Intervention PIIEF 6 months	9	
Control IIEF baseline	27	0.787**
Control PIIEF baseline	24	
Control IIEF 3 months	25	0.914**
Control PIIEF 3 months	22	
Control IIEF 6 months	22	0.725**
Control PIIEF 6 months	17	
Control IIEF 9 months	16	0.701*
Control PIIEF 9 months	12	

** Correlation is significant at the 0.01 level (2-tailed)   * Correlation is significant at the 0.05 level (2-tailed)

KEY ••••► Lifestyle changes ➡ Intervention ⟹ Home Exercises

Analysis of quality of life measurements

Table 5.10: Mean Erectile Dysfunction Effect on Quality of Life scores

Mean ED-EQoL scores	Intervention			Control Group			
Number of months from baseline	0	3	6	0	3	6	9
Sample number	28	25	17	27	25	22	16
1 Self-blame	2.3	1.9	1.9	2.8	2.4	2.5	2.1
2 Feelings of guilt	2.4	1.8	1.9	2.9	2.6	2.4	1.9
3 Feeling less desirable	2.0	1.6	1.2	2.1	2.2	2.0	1.9
4 Hurt by response of partner	1.2	0.6	1.0	1.4	0.8	1.1	1.1
5 Feeling less of a man	1.7	1.6	1.6	2.1	2.3	2.2	1.8
6 Feeling angry or bitter	1.5	1.5	1.1	2.3	2.3	2.4	1.6
7 Feel a failure	1.6	1.4	1.1	2.0	2.0	2.0	1.6
8 Partner feels let down	1.8	1.4	1.5	1.7	1.6	1.3	1.4
9 Affecting closeness with partner	1.5	1.3	1.5	1.6	1.8	1.4	1.2
10 Worry about future	1.6	1.6	1.5	2.3	1.8	1.5	1.6
11 Alteration in sense of identity	1.2	1.2	1.2	1.7	2.0	1.4	1.4
12 Preoccupation with erectile problems	1.4	1.2	0.9	1.7	1.6	1.4	1.2
13 Feeling of sadness	1.1	1.0	0.5	1.5	1.4	1.2	1.1
14 Feel other people are happier	1.5	1.5	1.4	2.1	1.9	1.7	1.6
15 Damage to self-esteem	1.7	1.2	1.5	1.9	1.8	1.5	1.4
Mean total (out of 60)	24.5	20.8	20.2	30.1	28.5	25.9	23.3

KEY
••••► Lifestyle changes ➡ Intervention ⟹ Home Exercises

There was a gradual decline in individual ED-EQoL scores for both the intervention and the control groups, indicating an improved quality of life for all subjects (Table 5.10). Possible individual total scores ranged from 60 (a great deal) to 0 (not at all). Each of the separate fifteen categories was ranked 4 (a great deal) to 0 (not at all). Questions 1, 2, and 3 (concerning 'self-blame', 'feelings of guilt' and 'feeling less desirable') were ranked more highly (worse) than other questions in both groups. Following intervention, subjects in both groups continued to score highly in 'self-blame' and 'feelings of guilt'.

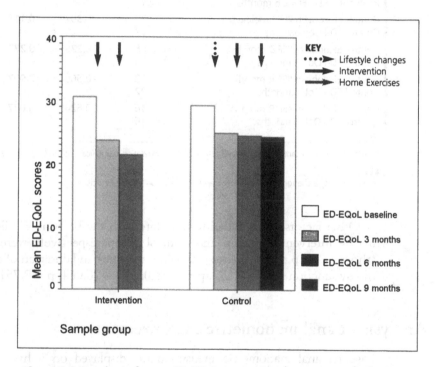

Figure 5.8: Bar chart of mean ED-EQoL scores at each assessment for intervention and control group

The mean scores of the ED-EQoL reduced as quality of life improved. In both groups there was improved quality of life at three months, but only minimal improvement in the control group following intervention and home exercises

There was poor correlation of the Erectile Function Domain of the IIEF with the ED-EQoL in both the intervention group and the control group (Table 5.11). There was correlation in the control group at six and nine months.

Table 5.11: Correlations of Erectile Function Domain of the IIEF and ED-EQoL for the intervention and control groups

Groups Compared	Number	Spearman's Correlation	Sig. (2-tailed)
Intervention EF domain IIEF baseline	28	–0.090	0.650
Intervention ED-EQoL baseline	28		
Intervention EF domain IIEF 3 months	25	–0.036	0.863
Intervention ED-EQoL 3 months	25		
Intervention EF domain IIEF 6 months	17	–0.216	0.405
Intervention ED-EQoL 6 months	17		
Control EF domain IIEF baseline	27	–0.307	0.119
Control ED-EQoL baseline	27		
Control EF domain IIEF 3 months	25	–0.228	0.273
Control ED-EQoL 3 months	25		
Control EF domain IIEF 6 months	22	–0.560**	0.007
Control ED-EQoL 6 months	22		
Control EF domain IIEF 9 months	16	–0.524*	0.037
Control ED-EQoL 9 months	16		

* Correlation is significant at the 0.05 level (2-tailed)   ** Correlation is significant at the 0.01 level (2-tailed)

KEY

••••▶ Lifestyle changes   ➡ Intervention   ➤ Home Exercises

Other factors which failed to correlate with the baseline ED-EQoL in the intervention group and control group respectively were age (rho = 0.016, p = 0.935) (rho = 0.034, p = 0.868) and duration of erectile dysfunction (rho = 0.337, p = 0.080) (rho = (0.064, p = 0.751).

Analysis of anal manometric measurements

Baseline anal manometric measurements displayed on a histogram showed an abnormal distribution curve, which was confirmed by a Kolmogorov-Smirnov test of normality allowing analysis by non-parametric tests. The mean scores for maximum anal pressure and anal hold pressure for the intervention group improved significantly at three months following intervention when compared to the control group using an independent Mann-Whitney U Test (p < 0.001) (Table 5.12).

At six months, in the intervention group there was no further significant improvement using a paired Wilcoxon Signed Ranks Test (Z = –1.256, p = 0.209). The control group failed to improve at three months with lifestyle changes (Z = –0.114, p = 0.909), but at six months following intervention they improved significantly (Z = –4.015, p < 0.001). There was no further improvement in the control group at nine months following home exercises when compared with six months using the same test (Z = –1.108, p = 0.268). The increases in maximum anal pressure measurements in Figure 5.9 mirrored the increases in the Erectile Function domain of the IIEF shown in Figure 5.5 for both groups.

Table 5.12: Results of unrelated Mann-Whitney Test for anal manometry at baseline and three months

Measurements	Group	No. of Men	Mean EF Domain	Range	U	Sig. (2-tailed)
Maximum pressure at baseline	Intervention	28	103.36	32–208	272.500	0.076
	Control	27	76.04	13–112		
Maximum pressure at 3 months	Intervention	25	147.52	51–242	36.500	< 0.001*
	Control	25	73.52	15–106		
Hold pressure At baseline	Intervention	28	92.39	38–196	278.000	0.092
	Control	27	70.37	11–112		
Hold pressure At 3 months	Intervention	25	133.68	49–235	37.500	< 0.001*
	Control	25	68.48	12–101		

* Denotes significant difference.

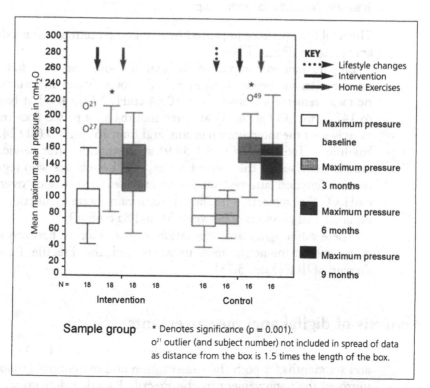

Figure 5.9: Boxplot of mean maximum anal pressure measurements at each assessment for both groups

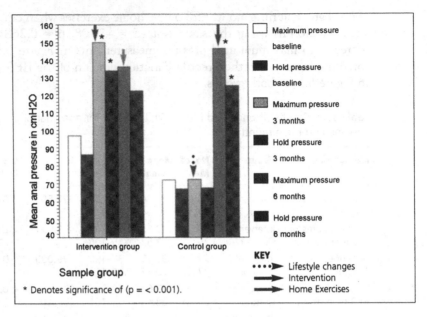

Figure 5.10: Bar chart of mean maximum and hold anal pressure at baseline, three and six months for both groups

The anal hold pressure improved in a similar pattern to the maximum anal pressure (Figure 5.10).

Erectile function improved as anal pressure improved following intervention and home exercises in both groups. Mean anal manometric measurements increased from 103.4 cmH_2O (SD 46.9) at baseline to 147.5 cmH_2O (SD 43.5) at three months after pelvic floor muscle exercises for the intervention group, and from 76 cmH_2O (SD 24.9) at baseline to 146.3 cmH_2O (SD 39.9) at six months after pelvic floor muscle exercises for the control group. All the subjects who regained normal function attained anal pressure measurements of over 100 cmH_2O. Six subjects who failed to regain normal function only attained anal pressures of between 51 and 85 cmH_2O.

There was a significant correlation at three months between maximum anal manometric measurements and the Erectile Function domain of IIEF (Table 5.13).

Analysis of digital anal measurements

The mean digital anal measurements were compared at baseline, three and six months for both the intervention and the control groups and mirrored the improvement in the Erectile Function domain scores of the IIEF and also the anal manometric measurements (Figure 5.11).

Table 5.13: Correlation of maximum anal manometric measurements with Erectile Function domain of IIEF for each assessment

Measurements	No. of Men	Spearman's	Significance (2-tailed)
Maximum anal pressure baseline Erectile Function domain IIEF baseline	55	0.232	0.089
Maximum anal pressure 3 months Erectile Function domain IIEF 3 months	50	0.366	0.009*
Maximum anal pressure 6 months Erectile Function domain IIEF 6 months	39	−0.007	0.967
Maximum anal pressure 9 months Erectile Function domain IIEF 9 months	16	0.387	0.139

* Denotes significant correlation.

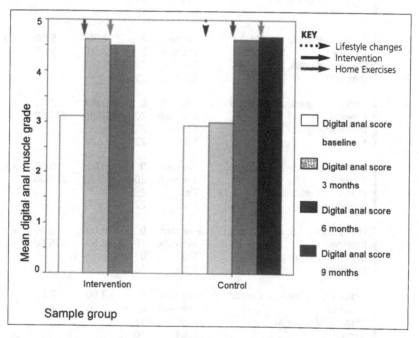

Figure 5.11: Bar chart of mean digital anal measurements at baseline, three and six months for both groups

Digital anal examination was compared in both groups for differences using a paired Wilcoxon test (Table 5.14). Results of this non-parametric test analysing ordinal data showed that all the groups improved significantly (p < 0.001) when compared to baseline except the control group at three months, and the intervention group and the control group receiving home exercises in the final three months of the trial.

Table 5.14: Results of digital anal examination for both groups

Paired Samples	Group	Ranks	No. of Men	Mean Rank	Sum of Ranks	Asymp. Sig. (2-tailed)
Digital anal grade at baseline Digital anal grade at 3 months	Intervention	−ve rank +ve rank Ties Total	2 2 21 25	2.50 2.50	5.00 5.00	< 0.001*
Digital anal grade at baseline Digital anal grade at 6 months	Intervention	−ve rank +ve rank Ties Total	0 15 3 18	0.00 8.00	0.00 120.00	0.001*
Digital anal grade at 3 months Digital anal grade at 6 months	Intervention	−ve rank +ve rank Ties Total	3 1 14 18	2.50 2.50	7.50 2.50	0.317
Digital anal grade at baseline Digital anal grade at 3 months	Control	−ve rank +ve rank Ties Total	2 2 21 25	2.50 2.50	5.00 5.00	1.000
Digital anal grade at baseline Digital anal grade at 6 months	Control	−ve rank +ve rank Ties Total	0 20 2 22	0.00 10.50	0.00 210.00	< 0.001*
Digital anal grade at 3 months Digital anal grade at 6 months	Control	−ve rank +ve rank Ties Total	0 20 2 22	0.00 10.50	0.00 210.00	< 0.001*
Digital anal grade at baseline Digital anal grade at 9 months	Control	−ve rank +ve rank Ties Total	0 16 0 16	0.00 8.50	0.00 136.00	< 0.001*
Digital anal grade at 6 months Digital anal grade at 9 months	Control	−ve rank +ve rank Ties Total	1 2 13 16	2.00 2.00	2.00 4.00	0.564

** Denotes significant difference.   KEY ••▶ Control ➡ Intervention ➡ Home Exercises

An overlay scatterplot of anal manometric measurements and digital anal grades showed positive correlation with a range of anal manometric readings for each digital anal examination grade (Figure 5.12).

There was a positive relationship between anal pressure scores and digital anal scores as shown in the scatterplot (Figure 5.12). However, a large range of maximum anal pressure readings equated to digital anal grade 5, which indicated a need for a digital anal grade 6 (very strong).

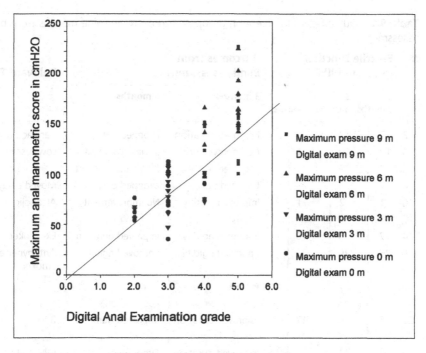

Figure 5.12: Scatterplot of digital anal grades and maximum anal manometric measurements at each assessment for both groups

Equally, there was significant correlation of maximum anal pressure with digital anal scores at baseline, three and six months, but not at nine months when using Spearman's correlation test (Table 5.15).

Table 5.15: Correlation of anal manometric measurements and digital anal grades for all subjects

Measurements	No. of Men	Spearman's
Maximum anal pressure scores at baseline	55	0.625**
Digital anal grades at baseline	55	
Maximum anal pressure scores at 3 months	50	0.835**
Digital anal grades at 3 months	50	
Maximum anal pressure scores at 6 months	40	0.556**
Digital anal grades at 6 months	40	
Maximum anal pressure scores at 9 months	16	0.336
Digital anal grades at 9 months	16	

** Correlation is significant at the 0.01 level (2-tailed).

Table 5.16: Outcomes of intervention group at three, six and nine months from blind assessment

N	Erectile Function Domain of IIEF			Outcomes from Blind Assessment		Relevant Factors
	0 months	3 months	6 months	3 months	6 months	
2	7	12	–	Improved duration	Dropped out	Cardiac bypass
4	13	10	4	No improvement	No improvement	Low testosterone
6	17	8	14	Improved rigidity	Improved duration	Normal function
8	7	–	–	Dropped out	Dropped out	Moved away
10	1	2	1	Improved rigidity	No improvement	Alcoholic
12	17	25	29	Improved duration	Normal function	
14	7	6	16	Improved rigidity	Improved duration	Ex-smoker
16	26	26	28	Improved rigidity	Improved rigidity	Anti-hypertensives; Smoker
18	8	27	29	Improved rigidity	Normal function	
20	28	30	–	Normal function	Dropped out	
22	5	9	17	Improved duration	Improved duration	BPH
24	24	29	29	Normal function	Normal function	
25	1	11	–	Improved duration	Dropped out	BPH and prostatitis
26	8	14	–	No improvement	Dropped out	Ex-smoker
28	6	29	24	Normal function	Normal function	
29	3	5	6	No improvement	No improvement	Cycle racer
31	1	26	25	Improved rigidity	Normal function	
32	4	28	28	Improved duration	Normal function	
35	15	13	12	Improved duration	Improved rigidity	Low testosterone
38	24	29	–	Normal function	Dropped out	Normal function
40	14	28	28	Injured	Normal function	Proctalgia and seepage better
41	6	6	–	No improvement	Dropped out	Diabetic
43	15	20	23	Improved duration	Improved duration	Diabetic
44	10	5	–	No improvement	Dropped out	Cardiovascular problems
48	1	22	29	Improved duration	Normal function	
50	2	–	–	Dropped out	Dropped out	Disliked anal probe
52	6	–	–	Dropped out	Dropped out	Normal function
53	18	11	–	Worse	Dropped out	Ex-smoker

Subjects with normal function outcome   KEY   ➤ Intervention   ➤ Home Exercises

0 m, 3 m and 6 m = Baseline, 3 months and 6 months assessments

Analysis of blind assessment results

The blind assessor completed the End of ED/PMD/Exit Questionnaire (Appendix 8). The erectile dysfunction scores from the blind assessment ranged from 0 = worse, 1 = same, 2 = some improvement in rigidity but not fully rigid, 3 = some improvement in duration but not fully rigid, to 4 = cured. There was good correlation between the Erectile Function domain of the IIEF and the blind assessments at three months from a Wilcoxon Signed Ranks test ($Z = -5.550$, $p = < 0.001$), six months ($Z = -5.137$, $p = < 0.001$) and nine months ($Z = -3.297$, $p = 0.001$).

Blind assessment of intervention group

Results from the blind assessment for the intervention group at six months showed that, including dropouts, twelve (42.9 per cent) men regained normal function, eight (28.6 per cent) improved and eight (28.6 per cent) failed to improve or dropped out (Tables 5.16 and 5.17). The data concerning subjects who had dropped out were taken from hospital notes by a registrar and from thank you letters. Of the subjects in the intervention group who had withdrawn by the end of the trial, three (10.7 per cent) regained normal function, two (7.1 per cent) improved, five (17.9 per cent) showed no improvement, while one (3.6 per cent) subject reported worsening erectile dysfunction (Table 5.17).

Table 5.17: Summary of outcomes of intervention group at three and six months from blind assessment

Outcomes of Intervention Group	Three Months' Intervention n = 28	Six Months' Home Exercises n = 28
Normal function	4 (14.3%)	9 (32.1%)
Improved duration	8 (28.6%)	3 (10.7%)
Improved rigidity	6 (21.4%)	3 (10.7%)
No improvement	6 (21.4%)	2 (7.1%)
Worse	1 (3.6%)	0
Dropped out – normal function	1 (3.6%)	3 (10.7%)
Dropped out – improvement	0	2 (7.1%)
Dropped out – no improvement	2 (7.1%)	5 (17.9%)
Dropped out – worse	0	1 (3.6%)
Total normal function including dropouts	5 (17.9%)	12 (42.9%)
Total improved including dropouts	14 (51.8%)	8 (28.6%)
Total with no improvement including dropouts	9 (32.1%)	8 (28.6%)

KEY ➡ Intervention ➡ Home Exercises

Table 5.18: Outcomes of control group at three, six and nine months from blind assessment

N	\multicolumn{4}{c}{Erectile Function Domain of IIEF}	\multicolumn{3}{c}{Outcomes from Blind Assessment}	Relevant Factors
	0 m	3 m	6 m	9 m	3 months control group	6 months control group	9 months control group	
1	11	4	–	–	No improvement	Dropped out	Dropped out	Ex-smoker
3	3	8	14	10	Improved rigidity	Improved duration	Improved duration	Peyronie's for surgery
5	5	5	5	–	No improvement	Dropped out	Dropped out	Diabetic LBP
7	16	2	26	12	Improved rigidity	Improved duration	No improvement	Low testosterone
9	11	5	23	23	No improvement	Improved rigidity	Normal function	–
11	8	1	20	–	Improved duration	Improved rigidity	Dropped out	Normal function
13	17	16	27	–	Improved rigidity	Normal function	Dropped out	–
15	17	12	29	28	Worse	Normal function	Normal function	–
17	5	1	20	20	No improvement	No improvement	Improved rigidity	Cardiac bypass
19	10	19	–	–	No improvement	Dropped out	Dropped out	Vasectomy pain
21	1	1	6	21	No improvement	No improvement	No improvement	Angina BP Smoker
23	6	6	18	30	No improvement	Improved rigidity	Improved duration	Beta blockers
27	1	1	1	1	No improvement	Improved rigidity	No improvement	Lack of libido
30	6	2	23	–	No improvement	Improved duration	Dropped out	No relationship
33	8	–	–	–	Dropped out	Dropped out	Dropped out	Abused as child
34	1	14	26	–	No improvement	Improved rigidity	Dropped out	Anti-hypertensives
36	3	3	15	12	No improvement	Improved rigidity	Improved rigidity	Beta blocker BP drugs
37	13	16	8	20	No improvement	Improved rigidity	Normal function	–
39	11	–	–	–	Dropped out	Dropped out	Dropped out	Normal function
42	12	23	29	29	Improved rigidity	Improved duration	Normal function	–
45	7	6	–	–	Improved rigidity	Dropped out	Dropped out	Alcoholic diabetic BP
46	9	15	29	28	No improvement	Improved rigidity	Normal function	–
47	1	1	5	–	No improvement	Improved duration	Dropped out	No relationship
49	6	9	19	14	No improvement	Improved rigidity	Improved rigidity	Pacemaker BP Smoker
51	4	16	12	15	No improvement	Improved rigidity	Improved rigidity	Orchidect's 30 years ED
54	4	1	20	20	No improvement	Improved rigidity	Normal function	–
55	15	22	27	28	Improved duration	Normal function	Normal function	–

Subjects with normal function outcome **KEY** ••▶ Lifestyle changes ➡ Intervention ➡ Home Exercises
0 m, 3 m and 6 m = Baseline, 3 months and 6 months assessments

Blind assessment of control group

Results from the blind assessment for the control group at nine months, showed that, including dropouts, ten (37 per cent) men regained normal function, eleven (40.7 per cent) improved and six (22.2 per cent) failed to improve or dropped out (Tables 5.18 and 5.19). Of the subjects in the control group who had withdrawn by the end of the trial, three (11.1 per cent) had regained normal function, five (18.5 per cent) improved and three subjects (11.1 per cent) showed no improvement (Table 5.19).

Table 5.19: Summary of outcomes of control group at three, six and nine months from blind assessment

Erectile Function Outcomes of Control Group	Three Months' Intervention n = 27	Six Months' Home Exercises n = 27	Nine Months' Intervention n = 27
Normal function	0	3 (11.1%)	7 (25.9%)
Improved duration	2 (7.4%)	5 (18.5%)	2 (7.4%)
Improved rigidity	5 (18.5%)	11 (40.7%)	4 (14.8%)
No improvement	17 (63.0%)	2 (7.4%)	3 (11.1%)
Worse	1 (3.7%)	0	0
Dropped out – normal function	1 (3.7%)	1 (3.7%)	3 (11.1%)
Dropped out – improvement	0	1 (3.7%)	5 (18.5%)
Dropped out – no improvement	1 (3.7%)	4 (14.8%)	3 (11.1%)
Dropped out – worse	0	0	0
Total normal function including dropouts	1 (3.7%)	4 (14.8%)	10 (37%)
Total improved including dropouts	7 (25.9%)	17 (63.0%)	11 (40.7%)
Total with no improvement including dropouts	19 (70.4%)	6 (22.2%)	6 (22.2%)

KEY   ••► Lifestyle changes   ➡ Intervention   ➡ Home Exercises

Number needed to treat

The number needed to treat (NNT) was calculated from the blind assessment outcomes of the randomised controlled trial at three months, by comparing the percentage of subjects attaining normal function including the drop outs in the intervention group (17.9 per cent) with those attaining normal function in the control group (3.7 per cent) (Tables 5.17 and 5.19).

$$NNT = \frac{100}{\% \text{ cured in intervention group} - \% \text{ cured in the control group}}$$

The number of subjects who needed to be treated to produce one additional successful outcome was calculated to be seven. This means that for one extra patient to attain normal function you need to treat seven subjects experiencing erectile dysfunction with pelvic floor muscle exercises instead of lifestyle changes. In this three-month period, the NNT required to achieve normal function *or improvement* with pelvic floor muscle exercises compared to the control group was three. Since few treatments are 100 per cent effective and few controls are without some effect, NNTs for very effective treatments are usually in the range of 2–4 (Moore and McQuay, 2002). This indicated that pelvic floor muscle exercises were a very effective treatment for the improvement of erectile dysfunction.

Combined groups blind assessment

The final analysis from the blind assessments of both groups combined including dropouts showed a total of 22 (40 per cent) subjects attained normal function, 19 (34.5 per cent) subjects had improved erectile function, while 14 (25.5 per cent) failed to improve (Table 5.20).

Table 5.20: Outcomes of both groups from blind assessment

Erectile Function Outcomes of Both Groups	After Three Months' Intervention n = 55 (100%)	After Three Months' Home Exercises n = 55 (100%)
Total normal function including dropouts	9 (16.4%)	22 (40.0%)
Total improved including dropouts	31 (56.4%)	19 (34.5%)
Total with no improvement including dropouts	15 (27.3%)	14 (25.5%)

At baseline, the subjects' appreciation of erectile dysfunction varied considerably from 1 to 28 points on the Erectile Function domain of the IIEF. Equally, subjects varied in their acceptance of normal function from 14 to 30 points (Table 5.21).

Table 5.21: Erectile Function domain of IIEF categories for those subjects who regained normal function

Erectile Function Score Category (Goldstein, 2000)	Baseline Score n = 21 (100%)	Normal Function Score n = 21 (100%)
No score	N/A	2 (9.5%)
Severe dysfunction (0–6)	6 (28.6%)	--
Moderate–severe dysfunction (7–12)	6 (28.6%)	--
Moderate dysfunction (13–18)	7 (33.3%)	1 (4.8%)
Mild dysfunction (19–24)	1 (4.8%)	5 (23.8%)
Normal function (25–30)	1 (4.8%)	13 (61.9%)

Analysis of lifestyle changes

The outcomes from changes of lifestyle were analysed separately for the intervention and control groups. No subject stopped smoking, most subjects reported an alcohol intake of two units a day or less, most men performed daily exercise such as hill walking or running up and down the stairs, some men lost weight and all the cyclists avoided sustained saddle pressure. The changes to lifestyle factors were similar in both groups. The control group who were undertaking three months of lifestyle changes only improved 0.76 points on the Erectile Function domain score of the IIEF during that period (see Table 5.4 above).

Linear regression analysis

Linear regression analysis was used in order to predict the individual risk factors such as age, duration of erectile dysfunction, smoking, alcoholic intake, anti-hypertensive medication, maximum and hold pelvic floor muscle strength which have an effect on erectile dysfunction at baseline. Natural logarithm was used on data from the dependent variable of the Erectile Function domain of the IIEF. There were no significant risk factors at baseline.

Table 5.22: Linear regression analysis of possible risk factors on Erectile Function domain of the IIEF at baseline

Variables	Beta Coefficient	Significance
Age	−0.149	0.366
Duration of erectile dysfunction	0.009	0.955
Smoker or ex-smoker	−0.055	0.727
Daily alcoholic intake	−0.031	0.838
Anti-hypertensive medication	−0.106	0.475
Maximum anal pressure at baseline	0.316	0.553
Anal hold pressure at baseline	−0.174	0.744
Digital anal measurements at baseline	−0.027	0.897

* Denotes significant correlation.

The same variables were individually analysed by linear regression analysis to determine whether the same risk factors had affected the Erectile Function domain of the IIEF at three months for the intervention group combined with the same domain at six months for the control group. Age was found to be significantly negatively correlated following intervention (β −0.418, p = 0.012) (Table 5.23). As there was no significant correlation between age with the Erectile Function domain at baseline, this indicated that it was possible to predict that younger men receiving pelvic floor exercises would have a better chance than older men of regaining erectile function. For every year of age, erectile function decreases by 0.418 points on the Erectile Function domain of the IIEF. Also, anti-hypertensive medication was found to be significantly negatively correlated following intervention (β –0.321, p = 0.027), which indicated that men performing pelvic floor muscle exercises who were not using anti-hypertensive medication would have a better chance of regaining erectile function.

Table 5.23: Linear regression analysis of possible risk factors on the Erectile Function domain for both groups following three months' intervention

Variables	Beta Coefficient	Significance
Age	–0.418	0.012*
Duration of erectile dysfunction	–0.005	0.974
Smoker or ex-smoker	–0.055	0.723
Daily alcoholic intake	–0.097	0.532
Anti-hypertensive medication	–0.321	0.027*
Maximum anal pressure at baseline	–0.269	0.606
Anal hold pressure at baseline	–0.139	0.788
Digital anal measurements at baseline	0.358	0.092

* Denotes significant correlation.

Analysis of covariance

One-way ANOVA (Analysis of Variance) was used to confirm or challenge the results of the Mann-Whitney independent samples test performed for a between-group difference in the Erectile Function domain of the IIEF at three months on 25 subjects (Table 5.24). The covariates used were subject group, age, body mass index, duration of erectile dysfunction, baseline Erectile Function domain of IIEF and baseline maximum anal pressure. Natural logarithms were used on the dependent variable.

The analysis of covariance confirmed the results of the Mann-Whitney independent samples test when controlling for the effect of other variable factors (Table 5.24). This analysis confirmed that pelvic floor muscle exercises and manometric biofeedback and lifestyle changes were significantly more effective than lifestyle changes.

Table 5.24: Analysis of covariance

Between-subject Factors	Value Label	Number of Subjects
Group 1	Intervention	25
Group 2	Control	25

Tests of Between-subject Effects
Dependent Variable: Erectile Function domain IIEF at 3 months

Source	F	Significance
Duration of erectile dysfunction	0.418	0.522
Age	1.721	0.197
Body Mass Index	0.277	0.601
Baseline Erectile Function domain IIEF	5.986	0.019*
Baseline maximum anal pressure	0.131	0.719
Intervention group	7.114	0.011*

Error df = 43

* Denotes significant difference.

Comparison of pelvic floor muscle exercises with sildenafil

The results of this trial were compared with a large grade II trial using oral sildenafil for 329 subjects with mixed aetiology (Goldstein et al., 1998). Both trials used the Erectile Function domain of the IIEF as the main outcome measure. In the trial by Goldstein et al. (1998), at twelve weeks subjects receiving up to 100 mg sildenafil based on efficacy and tolerance improved by ten points to attain a score of 21 points (Figure 5.13).

In the current trial, subjects in the intervention group improved at three months by eight points from the overall baseline score to attain a score of 17 points.

Conclusion

The intervention group showed a significant improvement (p = 0.001) in erectile function compared to the control group after three months with a clinical improvement of 6.74 points on the Erectile Function domain of the IIEF. The control group showed no significant increase in erectile function following lifestyle changes (p = 0.658), but a highly significant increase following intervention at six months (p < 0.001). There was clinical improvement of 9.88 points for the intervention

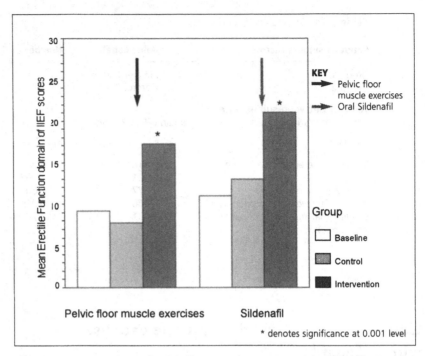

Figure 5.13: Comparison of pelvic floor muscle exercises with sildenafil using the Erectile Function domain of the IIEF

group and 10.94 points for the control group on the Erectile Function domain of the IIEF after three months of pelvic floor muscle exercises and three months of home exercises. There was, however, no significant improvement with home exercises in either the intervention group (p = 0.108) or control group (p = 0.646). There was good correlation between the IIEF and the PIIEF. The ED-EQoL correlated poorly with the Erectile Function Domain of the IIEF.

Manometric measurements and digital anal measurements showed that both groups improved significantly (p < 0.001) after intervention. Further improvement after home exercises was not significant. Subjects who regained normal function attained anal pressure measurements of 100 cmH$_2$O and above. Four subjects who failed to achieve anal pressure measurements in excess of 85 cmH$_2$O, showed no improvement. Anal manometric measurements were positively correlated with digital anal scales at baseline, three and six months (r > 0.556, p = 0.001). There was a need for another digital anal grade (grade 6, very strong) for assessing male pelvic floor musculature.

For all subjects after three months' intervention, 16.4 per cent regained normal function, 56.4 per cent improved, and 27.3 per cent failed to improve. After a further three months of home exercises, 40 per cent of subjects had attained normal function, 34.5 per cent had improved and 25.5 per cent failed to improve.

From the data it was also possible to predict that younger men receiving pelvic floor exercises would have a better chance than older men of regaining erectile function. It was also possible to predict that men receiving pelvic floor exercises who were not taking anti-hypertensive medication would have a better chance of regaining erectile function.

The results of this trial using pelvic floor muscle exercises for erectile dysfunction compared favourably with the results of a large grade II level evidence trial using oral sildenafil.

Chapter 6
Post-micturition dribble

Introduction

At the initial assessments, it was noted that many men reported post-micturition dribble. So, it was decided to undertake a critical appraisal of the literature and a detailed assessment of the current trial data to determine any effects of pelvic floor muscle exercises and manometric biofeedback on post-micturition dribble in this group.

Post-micturition dribble is the term used when an individual describes the involuntary loss of urine immediately after he has finished passing urine, usually after leaving the toilet (Abrams et al., 2002). It is neither stress-dependent nor due to bladder dysfunction (Wille et al., 2000) and should be distinguished from terminal dribble, which occurs at the end of micturition (Shah, 1994). Post-micturition dribble can be a nuisance and cause considerable embarrassment. It is common in all ages, including young men (Corcoran et al., 1987; Furuya et al., 1997), but is particularly troublesome in older men (Paterson et al., 1997). The prevalence of post-micturition dribble is reported to range from 11.5 to 63 per cent for men aged 20–70 years (Furuya et al., 1997; Koskimäki et al., 1998).

Aetiology

A number of causes have been suggested (Table 6.1). One functional cause that has been suggested is the failure of the bulbocavernosus muscle to evacuate urine from the bulbar portion of the urethra (Feneley, 1986; Millard, 1989). Rarer organic causes from congenital abnormalities and strictures have also been reported (Bullock, 2002). The treatment options vary and depend on the aetiology of post-micturition dribble (Table 6.1). Surgery is usually indicated for organic problems, while pelvic floor muscle exercises have been found to be effective for functional problems (Paterson et al. (1997).

Table 6.1: Aetiology and suggested treatment regimes for post-micturition dribble

Causes	Suggested Treatment	Reference
Pooling of urine in bulbous urethra	PFMEs Shake penis after voiding	Kondo et al. (2002)
Reduced or absent post-void milking reflex	PFMEs	Wille et al. (2000)
Bulbocavernosus muscle weakness	PFMEs	Paterson et al. (1997)
Urethral stricture	Surgery	Bullock (2002)
Congenital anterior urethral diverticulum	Surgery	Kondo et al. (2002)
Pressure from pants or high trouser zip on bulbar urethra	Drop underpants when urinating	Davies (1986) Furuya et al. (1997)

Critical appraisal of literature

In order to identify the prevalence, aetiology and treatment options for post-micturition dribble, a search was undertaken from the following computerised databases for the period 1980–2002: Medline, AAMED (Allied and Alternative Medicine), CINAHL, Nursing Collection, EMBASE – Rehabilitation and Physical Medicine and The Cochrane Library Database. The keywords chosen were 'post-micturition dribble, dribbling, post-void dribble, after-dribble, bulbocavernosus muscle, bulbar urethral massage, urethral milking and pelvic floor muscle exercises'. A manual search was undertaken of manuscripts found from the references of this literature.

All papers describing the prevalence, aetiology or treatment of post-micturition dribble were included in the review. Each paper was assessed for methodological rigour using the levels of evidence adapted from Sackett (1986) (see Table 2.1 above). The review revealed nine papers describing post-micturition dribble in men (Table 6.2) (Dorey, 2002). No level I evidence studies were found. Two papers provided level II evidence, six provided level III evidence and one provided only level V evidence (Table 6.2). Of these, three papers identified the prevalence of PMD from questionnaires and one described the action of the bulbocavernosus muscle during voiding cystourethrograms. One non-randomised controlled trial and two randomised controlled trials were found which explored the effect of pelvic floor muscle exercises on PMD. Two studies found an association between PMD and sexual dysfunction. Neither study explored reasons for this association. No

Table 6.2: Literature review of post-micturition dribble

Author/Design	Subjects	Method	Evidence	Outcomes
Malmsten et al. (1997) Sweden Random No control	7,763 men 45 years and older	Questionnaire	**Level III**	Prevalence of PMD 33.7 per cent men aged 45–90 years
Koskimäki et al. (1998) Finland Non-random No control	2,128 men aged 50, 60 and 70 years	Questionnaire	**Level III**	Prevalence of PMD 48 per cent mild 15 per cent moderate
Furuya et al. (1997) Japan Non-random No control	3,034 men aged 20–59 years	Questionnaire	**Level III**	Incidence of PMD 11.5 per cent aged 20–29 to 26.9 per cent aged 50–59
Wille et al. (2000) Switzerland No control Non-random	19 men	Voiding cysto-urethrograms pre- and post-radical prostatectomy	**Level V**	Pre-op twelve men had normal post-void milking Post-op one man had post-void milking
Chang et al. (1998) Taiwan Control Non-random	25 men PFMEs 25 men control	PFMEs after TURP for four weeks	**Level III**	At baseline 24 men with PMD in PFME group. At four weeks three men with PMD in PFME group
Porru et al. (2001) Italy Randomised Controlled	30 men in PFME group 28 men control	One pre-op PFMEs PFMEs post TURP for four weeks	**Level II**	PMD less in PFME group at one, two and three weeks No significant differ-ence at four weeks
Paterson et al. (1997) Australia Randomised Controlled	14 men PFMEs; 15 men milking 15 men counselling	PFMEs or Urethral milking or Counselling for 12 weeks	**Level II**	PFME group almost twice as effective as urethral milking Counselling no benefit
Frankel et al. (1998) UK Non-random No control	423 men in community 40 years+ 1,271 in clinic; 45 years+ in 12 countries	ICS 'BPH' study including ICS*male* & ICS*sex* questionnaires	**Level III**	Association between PMD and reduced rigidity 1.68 (p = 0.001) in clinic sample
Macfarlane et al. (1996) France Random No control	2,011 men 50–80 years	Survey	**Level III**	Association between PMD and sexual dys-function. Odds ratio 1.72 for moderate PMD, 2.20 for frequent PMD

Key:

PFMEs	=	pelvic floor muscle exercises	ICS	=	International Continence Society
TURP	=	transurethral resection of prostate,	BPH	=	benign prostatic hyperplasia

studies investigated the effect of pelvic floor muscle exercises on post-micturition dribble for men with erectile dysfunction.

One level II evidence study (Paterson et al., 1997) demonstrated a statistically significant mean loss of urine using pad tests in a group of men with post-micturition dribble receiving pelvic floor muscle exercises compared to a group receiving counselling (p = 0.001), but did not report the number of men who were identified by a clinician or by the men themselves as 'cured' or 'improved'. The other level II evidence trial (Porru et al., 2001) studied men following transurethral resection of prostate (TURP). The intervention group, which received one preoperative session of pelvic floor muscle exercises and post-operative pelvic floor muscle exercises, was compared with a control group. A significant reduction in post-micturition dribble was noted in the pelvic floor muscle group initially, but not at four weeks. Both studies indicated that pelvic floor muscle exercises had merit as a treatment for post-micturition dribble.

Results from current trial

Post-micturition dribble was self-reported by 21 (75 per cent) subjects in the intervention group, and 15 (55.6 per cent) in the control group at baseline, making a total of 36 (65.5 per cent) out of a sample of 55 men with erectile dysfunction (Table 6.3). In the intervention group, 14 (66.7 per cent) subjects at three months and 17 (81 per cent) subjects at six months reported no post-micturition dribble at the blind assessment. In the control group, following intervention, 9 (60 per cent) subjects at six months and 10 (67 per cent) subjects at nine months reported no post-micturition dribble at the blind assessment. For both groups combined, after intervention and home exercises, post-micturition dribble was reported at the blind assessment by only four (11.1 per cent) subjects. The results of a Wilcoxon Signed Ranks Test comparing each group with baseline showed significant improvement in both groups after intervention (Table 6.3). There was no significant improvement in the control group after three months' lifestyle changes.

In the two groups combined, after three months of pelvic floor muscle exercises and three months of home exercises, 27 (75 per cent) subjects were cured and reported no post-micturition dribble (Table 6.4) (Figure 6.1). Five (13.9 per cent) subjects had dropped out at this stage.

At baseline, post-micturition dribble was not correlated to age when analysed using Spearman's correlation (r = 0.129, p = 0.347). Also, using Spearman's correlation, no correlation was found between post-micturition dribble with the Erectile Function domain of the IIEF, manometric pressure and digital anal pressure at any assessment for either group.

Table 6.3: Frequencies of subjects with post-micturition dribble from the blind assessment

Sample	Group	PMD n (%)	Dropouts n (%)	Less Amount n (%)	Less Often n (%)	No PMD n (%)	Wilcoxon Test
Baseline	Intervention	21 (100%)	N/A	N/A	N/A	N/A	N/A
3 months	Intervention	2 (9.5%)	1 (4.8%)	2 (9.5%)	2 (9.5%)	14 (66.7%)	< 0.001*
6 months	Intervention	0	2 (9.5%)	1 (4.8%)	1 (4.8%)	17 (81.0%)	< 0.001*
Baseline	Control	15 (100%)	N/A	N/A	N/A	N/A	N/A
3 months	Control	10 (66.7%)	1 (6.7%)	1 (6.7%)	2 (13.3%)	1 (6.7%)	0.102
6 months	Control	2 (13.3%)	1 (6.7%)	0	3 (20.0%)	9 (60.0%)	0.001*
9 months	Control	1 (6.7%)	3 (20.0%)	0	1 (6.7%)	10 (67.0%)	0.002*

*   Asymptotic significance (2-tailed) based on Wilcoxon Signed Ranks Test

KEY
••••► Lifestyle changes ——► Intervention ——► Home Exercises

Table 6.4: Number of subjects from both groups with post-micturition dribble after three months' intervention and three months' home exercises

PMD at Baseline n (100 %)	Dropouts n (%)	PMD n (%)	Improved n (%)	Cured n (%)
36 (100%)	5 (13.9%)	1 (2.8%)	3 (8.3%)	27 (75.0%)

Number needed to treat

The number needed to treat (NNT) was calculated from the blind assessment outcomes of the randomised controlled trial at three months by comparing the percentage of subjects who were cured of post-micturition dribble in the intervention group (66.7 per cent) with those who were cured in the control group (6.7 per cent) (Table 6.3). At three months, the number of subjects who needed to be treated (NNT) to produce one additional subject cured of post-micturition dribble was caculated to be two. In the same time frame, the percentage of subjects who were cured or improved in the intervention group (85.7 per cent) was compared with the percentage of subjects who were cured or improved in the control group (26.7 per cent) (Table 6.3). At three months, the NNT to produce one additional subject cured or improved of post-micturition dribble was also calculated to be two.

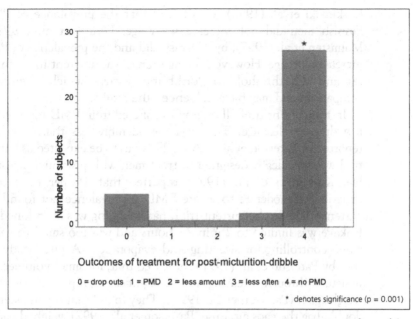

Figure 6.1: Bar chart of post-micturition dribble treatment outcomes after pelvic floor muscle exercises and home exercises for both groups combined

Discussion

A key finding in this study was the large percentage of men with erectile dysfunction who also experienced post-micturition dribble (65.5 per cent). This incidence was greater in men with erectile dysfunction than in other studies, in which the incidence of erectile dysfunction is unknown. Other studies have reported an incidence of 11.5 per cent to 26.9 per cent (Furuya et al., 1997), 33.7 per cent (Malmsten et al., 1997) and 63 per cent (Koskimäki et al., 1998). However, Koskimäki et al. (1998) reported that the answers may have included two types of dribbling – terminal and post-micturition – and Malmsten et al. (1997) simply reported 'dribbling', which may have included both types. The incidence reported by Furuya et al. (1997) may be more realistic, especially as their questionnaire was post-micturition dribble-specific and not related to a range of lower urinary tract symptoms. The prevalence of post-micturition dribble remains unknown, but it appears to be more prevalent in men with erectile dysfunction. There may be many factors preventing men from acknowledging the problem: embarrassment, a wish to be independent, a belief that it is normal or part of ageing, and lack of knowledge of the effectiveness of conservative treatments.

In the current study, post-micturition dribble was not correlated with age at baseline (r = 0.129, p = 0.347), which confirmed the findings of

Koskimäki et al. (1998), who found that the prevalence of PMD in Finnish men did not increase with age. Furuya et al. (1997) and Malmsten et al. (1997), by contrast, did find the prevalence of PMD to increase with age. However, the age range was different in all the studies and the threshold of 'dribbling' varied, which compromised comparison and may have influenced the results.

In the current trial all men who suffered from PMD reported just a few drops of leakage. This was considerably less than the leakage reported by Paterson et al. (1997). This was to be expected as Paterson's trial was specifically designed to treat men with post-micturition dribble. Koskimäki et al. (1998) reported that 15 per cent of men experienced moderate to severe PMD, a prevalence not found in the current study. In the current trial, pad weighing was abandoned as the leakage was limited to 2 g in 24 hours and was too small to calculate when controlling for sweating and evaporation. A pilot study in the trial by Paterson et al. (1997) indicated that, for small volumes, added moisture through sweating was a significant proportion of the pad weight gain (Paterson et al., 1997). They found that it was essential to double-bag the pads after use. Paterson et al. (1997) weighed pads after four hours' use and found most patients experienced losses of < 15 g at the beginning of the study, with some men having losses of > 20 g. This trial failed to report the amount of leakage following each void. There was no information concerning the number of voids in four hours, although the trial did show that men with larger initial losses tended to make greater improvement. However, if the initial loss had been small, it may not have been possible to detect a treatment effect. In this group of fourteen men, the mean data may have been skewed because the group contained a few men with large initial losses who improved dramatically. The number of visits to the therapist was not stated nor, more importantly, was the number of men who were cured.

In the current study, in both groups some subjects improved after three months' intervention, while others improved after three months of home exercises (Table 6.3). There was a high success rate in relieving post-micturition dribble using pelvic floor muscle exercises (75 per cent) (Figure 6.1). This confirmed the findings in Paterson et al.'s (1997) level II evidence trial. They showed, in 43 men who completed the programme, that pelvic floor exercises were almost twice as likely to have reduced urine loss (4.7 g) than urethral milking (bulbar urethral massage) (2.9 g). These results were not statistically significant, but treatment by either method was more effective than counselling alone (p = 0.001).

In the current trial, the low NNTs indicated that pelvic floor muscle exercises that included a post-void 'squeeze-out' muscle contraction (see Chapter 2) over a three-month period were very effective for the cure and improvement of post-micturition dribble in men with erectile dysfunction. This improvement may have been due to strengthening the pelvic floor musculature or to the functional 'squeeze-out' muscle contraction performed after voiding, which replaced the reduced or absent bulbocavernosus reflex.

During my work as a continence specialist physiotherapist, I found that patients with post-micturition dribble, who performed a strong voluntary pelvic floor muscle contraction after the completion of voiding, were able to eject a few more drops of urine. On the basis of this clinical experience, development of this skill has been encouraged. In order to investigate the effect of a pelvic floor muscle contraction immediately after voiding, a visit was arranged to the Urodynamics Department at Southmead Hospital, Bristol to watch a videocystourethrogram. One patient, who suffered from post-micturition dribble, was requested to 'tighten his pelvic floor muscles strongly as if to prevent the flow of urine' immediately after voiding. This voluntary post-void 'squeeze-out' was seen to eject opaque medium from the bulbar urethra. An oblique videourethrogram taken prior to the 'squeeze-out' contraction showed urine in the bulbar urethra (Figure 6.2) and another videourethrogram during the voluntary 'squeeze-out' contraction showed the bulbar urethra to be empty (Figure 6.3). These findings led to the exploration of possible explanations for the effectiveness of pelvic floor muscle exercises for post-micturition dribble and a possible association between post-micturition dribble and erectile dysfunction.

The contraction seen during the videocystogram may be explained by Wille et al.'s (2000) results. They postulated that the bulbocavernosus and ischiocavernosus muscles may be involved in clearing the urethra at the end of normal voiding. They described an antegrade wave from the external urethral sphincter through the urethra at the end of voiding which cleared the urethra of urine in 63 per cent of preoperative voiding cystourethrograms. They found that the efferent nerve supply via the pudendal nerve to the bulbocavernosus and ischiocavernosus muscles was untouched during radical prostatectomy and therefore loss of post-void urethral milking should not be due to interruption of the motor pathway. They suggested that a possible reason was damage to the sensory innervation of the external urethral sphincter. Recent investigations have shown a decrease in sensitivity in the membranous urethra after pelvic surgery (Hugonnet et al., 1999). This may be due to surgical trauma or the presence of a catheter. This would indicate the importance of sensory as well as motor innervation to maintain continence (Wille et al., 2000).

Another possibility is post-surgical pain, which could render the bulbocavernosus muscle inactive or ineffective. Wille et al. (2000) also

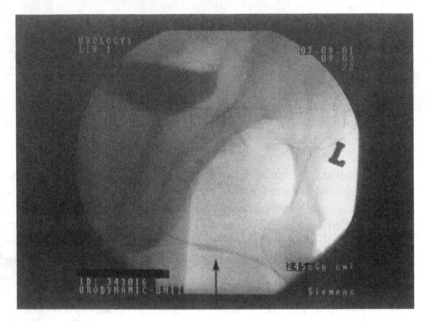

Retained urine

Figure 6.2: Videograph showing bulbar urethra before 'squeeze out' muscle contraction

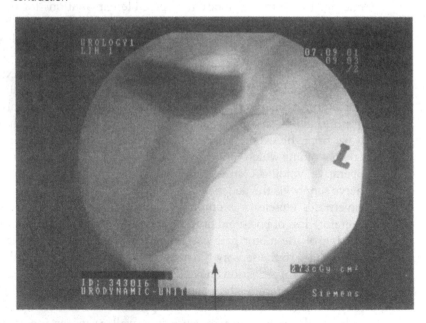

Catheter line showing but no retained urine

Figure 6.3: Videograph of man in Figure 6.2 during 'squeeze out' muscle contraction eliminating urine from bulbar urethra

suggested that benign prostatic hyperplasia may be responsible for a reduced or absent post-void milking reflex. Stephenson and Farrar (1977) used urodynamics to demonstrate a milk-back of contrast medium from the prostatic urethra to the bladder during voluntary interruption of the urine stream.

Shafik and El-Sibai (2000a) studied fourteen healthy male volunteers to test the response of bulbocavernosus muscle to urethral distension. They found that distension of between 0.5 ml and 1.5 ml caused increased EMG activity of the bulbocavernosus muscle. They concluded that this bulbocavernosus contraction was probably mediated through the urethrocavernosus reflex. This reflex is important for ejaculation, but it may also play a part in eliminating urine following micturition.

During cystometry, Vereecken and Verduyn (1970) observed a transient perineal contraction accompanied by a urethral pressure peak at the end of voiding, which was accompanied by a visible contraction of the bulbocavernosus muscle and tended to expel the last drops of urine from the urethra.

The pelvic floor muscle regime varied in each trial, which compromised comparisons. In the current trial, pelvic floor muscle exercises were taught in lying, sitting and standing positions, with a 50 per cent lift while walking occasionally and a post-void 'squeeze-out' muscle contraction (Appendix 6). Subjects were instructed to tighten and lift as if interrupting the flow of urine and observe a penile retraction and scrotal lift. Paterson et al. (1997) and Porru et al. (2001) used a similar regime, but included no 50 per cent lift in walking for muscle endurance and no functional post-void muscle contraction. In the trial conducted by Porru et al. (2001), subjects practised a total of 45 exercises (the number of exercise sessions was not stated in the trial by Paterson et al., 1997). In the current trial subjects performed fewer exercises; instead emphasis was placed on producing maximum strength for each contraction in order to achieve muscle strengthening (see Chapter 2). It may be that the voluntary 'squeeze-out' muscle contraction helped to evacuate urine from the bulbar urethra, and replaced or possibly developed the reflex post-void milking mechanism identified by Wille et al. (2000). (Shafik and El-Sibai (2000a) call this the urethrocavernosus reflex). It was hypothesised that the urinary sphincter contracted with the pelvic floor muscles, but this action has not been identified.

Manometric biofeedback was used in the current trial to motivate subjects and enhance performance. No trials were found in the literature, which used anal manometry in the treatment of post-micturition dribble. It was impossible to know whether this biofeedback had enhanced the results.

In the current trial, outcomes were self-reported to the blind assessor who completed the 'End of ED/PMD Study/Exit Questionnaire' at
the three-, six- and nine-month assessments (Appendix 8). Categories
for the self-reported outcomes at the blind assessment were 'Worse',
'Same', 'Less amount of leakage', 'Less amount of leakage and less
often', and 'Cured'. After three months' intervention and three
months' home exercises, all subjects reported to the clinician that they
were experiencing no post-micturition dribble (i.e. were cured), though
four reported some after-dribble to the blind assessor. These subjects
could 'squeeze out' a little more urine after voiding and experienced no
PMD at this stage. It is possible that they misled the blind assessor by
reporting the urine loss that occurred during the 'squeeze-out' muscle
contraction as 'after-dribble'. No other trial has included a specific post-
void 'squeeze-out' contraction with pelvic floor muscle exercises. There
is an analogy between the functional 'squeeze-out' muscle contraction
and the pelvic floor muscle contraction known as 'the knack' (Miller et
al., 1996).

'The knack' is a method of voluntarily contracting the pelvic floor
muscles just before and during activities that increase the intra-abdominal pressure. It replaces or reinforces the normal guarding reflex of the
external urethral sphincter. The 'squeeze-out' muscle contraction also
replaces or reinforces the normal bulbocavernosus reflex.

Association between post-micturition dribble and erectile dysfunction

Data from the current trial indicated that post-micturition dribble was
a common complaint in men suffering from erectile dysfunction. Two
studies have shown an association between PMD and sexual dysfunction, although neither study suggested a reason for this. In a study of
men aged 45 years and over conducted in twelve countries, Frankel et
al. (1998) showed that there was a significant association between
PMD and erectile dysfunction among symptomatic clinic attenders
(odds ratio 1.68, $p = < 0.001$). Macfarlane et al. (1996) found in men
between 50 and 80 years of age in the community that the odds ratio
for an association between PMD and sexual dysfunction was 1.72 for
moderate dribbling and 2.20 for frequent dribbling.

In the current trial, pelvic floor muscle exercises have been shown
to have merit for the treatment of both erectile dysfunction and post-
micturition dribble. Pelvic floor muscle exercises could be used to
prevent or reverse muscle weakness caused by disuse and may help to
restore functional use of these muscles.

It has been shown that contraction or reflex contraction of the ischiocavernosus and bulbocavernosus muscles produced an increase in the intracavernous pressure in the tumescent penis (Lavoisier et al., 1986). It has also been demonstrated that the bulbocavernosus muscle acted as a suction-ejection pump to propel the semen down the urethra resulting in ejaculation (Shafik and El-Sibai, 2000a). In the current study, in response to IIEF question 9 ('*Over the past four weeks, when you had sexual stimulation or intercourse, how often did you ejaculate?*'), the frequency of ejaculation improved from baseline in the intervention group following three months' pelvic floor muscle strengthening (p = 0.035) compared to the control group (p = 0.705) (Table 5.4). Weak ischiocavernosus and bulbocavernosus muscles may be unable to produce an increase in the intracavernous pressure. Similarly, a loss of ejaculation force was probably caused by loss of rhythmic contractions of the bulbocavernosus muscle (Shafik and El-Sibai, 2000b). Post-micturition dribble was attributed to a failure of the bulbocavernosus muscle to evacuate the bulbar portion of the urethra (Feneley, 1986; Millard, 1989). Wille et al. (2000) postulated that the bulbocavernosus and ischiocavernosus muscles were involved in clearing the urethra at the end of normal voiding. Shafik and El-Sibai (2000a) reported that a bulbocavernosus contraction was probably mediated through the urethrocavernosus reflex. Whereas this reflex is important for ejaculation, it may also play a part in eliminating urine following micturition.

Yang and Bradley (1999) found that electrical stimulation to the anterior urethra caused a bulbocavernosus muscle contraction, suggesting that the somatic afferents from the anterior urethra were involved in the ejaculatory reflex. Yang and Bradley (2000) recorded three distinct somatic bulbocavernosus reflexes. Bulbocavernosus muscle contraction was elicited after stimulating the dorsal nerve at the glans and anterior urethra by flexor responses of the bulbocavernosus reflex. Bulbocavernosus muscle contraction can also be induced on stimulating the perineal nerve, which is the pathway through which stretch and tendon organ reflexes are carried to mediate muscle tone. The bulbocavernosus reflex therefore depends on sensory afferents from the dorsal and perineal nerves, the conus medullaris and motor efferents via the perineal nerve. As the motor innervation of the bulbocavernosus muscle for all reflexes is carried through a branch of the perineal nerve, these findings may be relevant to the evaluation of ejaculatory disorders and post-micturition dribble.

The bulbocavernosus muscle, therefore, is active in post-void elimination of urine, penile rigidity and ejaculation of semen. Bulbocavernosus muscle dysfunction may cause a loss of the post-void milking reflex, an inability to produce an increase in intracavernous pressure and a loss of ejaculation force. Bulbocavernosus muscle dysfunction may explain the association between erectile dysfunction and post-micturition dribble. It may explain the reason for the increased prevalence of post-micturition dribble among men with erectile dysfunction. Pelvic floor muscle exercises may help to improve and prevent both these conditions.

Conclusion

Post-micturition dribble is a common condition. The overall prevalence remains unknown, but it is associated with erectile dysfunction. In the current trial, post-micturition dribble was present in 65.5 per cent of subjects with erectile dysfunction at baseline, which was greater than in other studies for men with a similar age range. In the current trial, post-micturition dribble was not correlated with age, which was in line with one study but disagreed with two other studies.

Of the 36 subjects who completed three months of pelvic floor muscle exercises and three months of home exercises, 27 (75 per cent) who experienced PMD at baseline were cured, three (8.3 per cent) improved, five (13.9 per cent) dropped out and one (2.8 per cent) continued to experience leakage.

From the current trial, pelvic floor muscle exercises including a 'squeeze-out' muscle contraction have been shown to be an effective treatment for post-micturition dribble in men with erectile difficulties. The cure rate using this method of treatment in 36 men was shown to be 75 per cent ($p = 0.001$).

The bulbocavernosus muscle is active in post-void elimination of urine, penile rigidity and ejaculation of semen. Bulbocavernosus muscle dysfunction may explain the association between erectile dysfunction and post-micturition dribble.

Chapter 7
Discussion

Analysis of outcome measures for erectile dysfunction

Erectile Function domain of the IIEF

Measurement by the main outcome measure, the Erectile Function domain of the IIEF, indicated that there was both significant and clinical improvement in the intervention group at three months compared to the control group. This was the first randomised controlled trial to use a validated outcome to measure the effectiveness of pelvic floor muscle exercises enhanced by manometric biofeedback. This result was in line with non-randomised or uncontrolled trials, which have also shown improvement with these treatment modalities. The control group failed to improve in the first three months with lifestyle changes, but improved following treatment with pelvic floor muscle exercises and biofeedback for three months. Both groups then showed a slower rate of improvement after a further three-month period performing a home regime of pelvic floor muscle exercises.

All the subjects had experienced erectile dysfunction for six months or more prior to participation in the trial, which was in line with the medical history warranting treatment, as suggested by Cappelleri and Rosen (1999). There was a surprisingly wide variation between subjects of what constituted erectile dysfunction as measured by the Erectile Function domain of the IIEF. Baseline scores of the Erectile Function domain of the IIEF ranged from 1 to 28 points. Similarly, there was a wide variation in the Erectile Function domain scores of the subjects who reported normal function at the blind assessment, with scores ranging from 14 to 30 points. This was not in line with the categories of the Erectile Function domain used by Goldstein (2000) and suggests a wide variation in what is considered normal function. It may be that this domain of the IIEF fails to address the range of perceived normal function, or it may be that subjects who had attained normal function but had not performed sexual activity in the month prior to completing the

103

questionnaire gave low scores. One subject with a partner at baseline and a score of 17 points scored only 14 points at the final assessment even though he regained normal function as he no longer had a partner and therefore returned scores of zero (i.e. did not attempt intercourse) for questions 3, 4 and 5. The severity categories suggested by Albaugh and Lewis (1999), which ranked satisfactory erection attempts out of ten, might have been a more realistic indicator (see Table 1.1, p. 1). This classification included men who self-stimulated and men who preferred sexual activity without vaginal penetration. A more realistic solution could be to rephrase questions 3, 4 and 5 of the IIEF to address men without a relationship, those who preferred non-vaginal sexual activity and those who preferred to self-stimulate. For example, question 3 could be changed to read: 'Over the past four weeks, when you attempted sexual intercourse (sexual acitivity or masturbated), how often were you able to penetrate your partner (or achieve satisfactory stimulation or self-stimulation)?' Similarly, for all questions, 'Over the past four weeks' could be changed to: 'Over the past four weeks (or when you last had sexual activity)' in line with the IIEF-5, in order to target those men unable to perform in that time frame for whatever reason. The reasons included: 'My wife had a bad back', 'My wife went to look after her parents', 'I slipped on the ice and fractured two ribs', 'I had a serious car accident' and 'I fell off a ladder'.

Interestingly, only one man who regained normal erectile function responded to IIEF question 15, 'How do you rate your confidence that you can get and keep your erection?', with a score of 5 (Very high). This may have indicated that even when men regained normal function they still lacked confidence or feared a recurrence of former erectile difficulties.

Examination of individual cases revealed the return of self-reported nocturnal erections following 1–4 weeks of pelvic floor muscle exercises and prior to regaining erectile function. This was in line with Lavoisier et al.'s (1988) study. They demonstrated that contractions of the perineal muscles strongly coincided with changes in penile rigidity during nocturnal erections ($p < 0.001$). It seems reasonable to suggest that increased strength in the pelvic floor muscles would improve the muscular phase responsible for increasing penile rigidity.

Results showed that ejaculatory function also improved with pelvic floor muscle exercises. In answer to IIEF question 9 regarding frequency of ejaculation, there was significant improvement at three months in the intervention group ($p = 0.035$), but no improvement in the control group ($p = 0.705$) (see Table 5.4 above). This is not surprising as the bulbocavernosus muscle, which pumps the ejaculate, would have been strengthened along with the other pelvic floor muscles. This supports Shafik and El-Sibai (2000a), who found that bulbocavernosus muscle weakness caused a loss of ejaculation force.

There was good evidence of a correlation between the IIEF and the PIIEF, which possibly indicated and reinforced the accuracy of the subjects' responses in the IIEF, although partners could have conferred with the subjects while completing the PIIEF. However, it was designed to give an opportunity to involve partners, even though this was at the discretion of the subjects. It was a failure of the IIEF that it did not provide any specific information about the relationship or sexual function of the partner (Rosen et al., 2002). At baseline, 23 (82.1 per cent) partners of men in the intervention group and 24 (88.9 per cent) partners of men in the control group completed the PIIEF. This indicated a willingness on the part of most partners to be involved in the treatment process, even though only five (9 per cent) had instigated the referral process. Many studies of the treatment of erectile dysfunction failed to mention any partner involvement (Schouman and Lacroix, 1991; Claes and Baert, 1993; Claes et al., 1995; Colpi et al., 1999). There is increasing recognition that the partner should be involved in the assessment, diagnosis, patient education, counselling and choice of treatment for treatment to be successful (Hawton, 1998). Nehra et al. (2002) recognised that men and their partners needed to be educated and counselled to achieve satisfactory sex, with treatment encompassing the relationship.

In the intervention group two men had no partner. Two men dropped out of the control group before the nine-month assessment because their relationships had failed. Many patients not in a relationship are reluctant to embark on one as they fear erectile failure (Dinsmore and Evans, 1999).

The literature suggests that various factors would have an effect on the severity of erectile dysfunction. Some men reported that their symptoms had commenced after taking anti-hypertensive medication. Indeed, this medication seemed to have a negative effect on erectile function following three months of pelvic floor muscle exercises. It was a surprise to find that age, duration of erectile dysfunction, alcohol, smoking and body mass index correlated poorly with the Erectile Function domain of the IIEF at baseline. Following intervention, it was unexpected to find that age was a factor that correlated with the same domain for both groups. The impact of age was understandable as younger men may well have fewer co-morbidities, be generally fitter and more able to cope with a muscle strengthening regime.

ED-EQoL

As erectile function improved, quality of life also improved slightly at each assessment. Despite this, results showed poor correlation of the IIEF with the ED-EQoL in the intervention group, but significant correlation in the control group. It may have been that the quality of life of the subjects in the control group was more closely related to all aspects of sexual function than the intervention group or, conversely, the correlation may have been due purely to chance. More importantly, the Erectile Function domain of the IIEF showed poor correlation with the ED-EQoL in both groups. These results were similar to MacDonagh et al.'s (2002). They found reasonable correlation with the satisfaction domains of the IIEF, but lack of correlation with aspects relating to the severity of erectile function. They concluded that it was difficult to achieve high correlations when one of the variables had a narrow range of scores. However, in this trial the range of scores in the Erectile Function domain was large. This shows that erectile dysfunction may have impacted on men in different ways, for example hormonal influences, relationship issues, increasing age or cultural and religious influences, and may explain why some men demonstrated considerable anxiety while others appeared not to be particularly bothered, although they were concerned enough to present for treatment. Subjects in both groups scored more highly (worse) at each assessment in response to question 1 'Do you blame yourself for being unable to satisfy your partner?' and question 2 'Does your inability to produce an erection with your partner make you feel guilty?' 'Self-blame' and feelings of 'guilt' may raise the need for counselling. These influences may explain why age and duration of erectile dysfunction failed to correlate with the ED-EQoL at baseline. These poor correlations perhaps demonstrated a clear reason for the clinical usefulness of a quality of life questionnaire such as the ED-EQoL in the treatment of men with erectile problems.

The scoring system of the ED-EQoL would be more meaningful if it ranged from 0 (worst) to 60 (best) as quality of life increased, instead of the reverse. This would be in line with the scoring system for the IIEF, which ranges from 0 (poor erectile function) and increases to 75 (normal erectile function).

Anal manometric measurements

In the trial, all subjects reported completion of their home exercise regime to the clinician and most subjects showed a substantial improvement on both digital anal and anal manometric measurements, even though some subjects failed to regain erectile function. This compliance was much better than the exercise performance rates in other trials. Claes et al. (1995) reported that some of the subjects failed to perform home exercises, while Colpi et al. (1994) reported that 11 out of 33 (33.3 per cent) failed to perform their pelvic floor exercises.

All men were able to achieve a penile retraction and scrotal lift during training with pelvic floor muscle exercises, though this was often difficult and slow initially. As muscle strength improved, the response was initiated at a faster rate. Subjects found it easier to achieve a scrotal lift in lying than against gravity in standing. Men who had a varicocoele found the scrotal lift sluggish initially on the affected side.

Mean anal manometric measurements in both groups increased from 89.7 cmH$_2$O at baseline to 146.9 cmH$_2$O after three months of pelvic floor muscle exercises. Four subjects who had low anal pressure measurements after intervention (51–85 cmH$_2$O) remained weak and failed to achieve normal function, giving added weight to the argument that weak pelvic floor muscles were a risk factor for erectile dysfunction.

Anal manometric measurements correlated well with the Erectile Function domain of the IIEF at three months, showing that subjects with weaker pelvic floor muscles experienced more severe dysfunction. This confirmed Colpi et al.'s (1999) study, which found significantly higher EMG measurements in normal men than in men with erectile dysfunction. This was the first time that anal manometric measurements have been used as an outcome measure for pelvic floor muscle strength in men with erectile dysfunction. For both groups, after three months of pelvic floor muscle exercises and three months of home exercises, the anal manometric measurements failed to correlate with the Erectile Function domain of the IIEF assessment at that time. This could be because most men attained considerable improvement in pelvic floor muscle strength irrespective of whether erectile function returned. This finding confirmed that men with erectile dysfunction entering the trial had weak pelvic floor musculature. This weakness appears to be associated with erectile dysfunction.

Digital anal measurements

Results have shown that digital anal examination grades correlated significantly with anal manometric measurements. However, at nine months they failed to correlate. This may be due to the high manometric pressures achieved by men following pelvic floor muscle training, which could only be graded 5 (strong), by digital anal examination. In the only other study comparing manometry with digital examination, Haslam (1999) found good correlation between vaginal manometry and digital vaginal examination ($r = 0.619$, $p < 0.05$). However, this was not directly comparable to anal measurements. We saw in Chapter 4 that reliable clinical measurements of anal pressure could be obtained in a group of men with erectile difficulties. This would indicate that for men anal manometry with a ratio level of measurement is more accurate than using five grades of ordinal level of measurement during digital anal examination. Fynes et al. (1999) studied a group of women and found after pelvic floor muscle strengthening anal maximum squeeze pressures of 101 mmHg, equivalent to 74.2 cmH_2O, which were considerably less than the anal pressure measurements in men. Figure 5.17 shows that the range of manometric scores graded 5 digitally range from 92 cmH_2O to 225 cmH_2O. It may be that for digital anal assessment in men, grade 6 (very strong) is needed.

Blind assessment

The blind assessment indicated that out of 55 subjects, 40 per cent regained normal erectile function, 34.5 per cent improved and 25.5 per cent failed to improve. Of the subjects who dropped out, six (10.9 per cent) had regained normal function, seven (12.7 per cent) had improved, eight (14.5 per cent) had failed to improve and one (1.8 per cent) experienced more severe erectile dysfunction. These results are in line with previous studies using pelvic floor muscle exercises, which either lacked randomisation or controls, or both, and reported that 46 per cent (Van Kampen et al., 1998), 26 per cent (Claes et al., 1996b) 36 per cent (Claes et al., 1995) and 42 per cent (Claes and Baert, 1993) of men regained normal function. A randomised controlled trial often yields poorer results due to the methodological rigour used to eliminate bias, but results were comparable with other studies despite the differences of selection criteria, subject age and duration of erectile dysfunction.

Many subjects willingly attended the blind assessment with the urologist (or his registrar) and were grateful to be given the opportunity to discuss urological problems. However, a few refused to make an appointment, as they felt that this would not be of direct benefit to their problem. Therefore, some blind assessments were undertaken by the specialist nurse at the erectile dyfunction clinic, some data were gleaned from patient notes and for three subjects reporting normal function, the data were taken from thank-you letters. It would have been easier if there had been a blind assessor in the physiotherapy department, who could have seen patients directly before their assessments. It was not necessary for the blind assessor to have medical experience. The ability to record the data impartially on the 'End of ED/PMD Study Exit Questionnaire' form (Appendix 8) was sufficient.

There was good correlation between the blind assessments and the Erectile Function domain of the IIEF at three, six and nine months, which further reinforced the results from the main outcome measure.

Analysis of subjects who dropped out

In the current trial, 22 (40 per cent) subjects did not remain for the planned duration. Of these, six (10.9 per cent) withdrew because they had achieved normal erectile function and seven (12.7 per cent) withdrew following improved erectile function. Nine (16.4 per cent) subjects withdrew showing no improvement. The number of subjects who dropped out was a concern to the researcher, even though Nehra et al. (2002) reported a high discontinuation rate in patients undergoing treatment for erectile dysfunction. In the current trial, one of the most frequent reasons reported was that the subject regained normal function. While the researcher was pleased with the result, the importance of the three- and six-month assessments had been explained to them. However, many men were adamant that they wished to withdraw and their request and sensibilities were respected. The researcher was constantly aware of the embarrassment suffered by this cohort. Those men who were not improving requested alternative treatment and were referred to the erectile dysfunction clinic. Initially, many of the men had presented to the urologist with the expectation of obtaining sildenafil and were diverted into the current trial. According to MacDonagh et al. (2002), many men seek a quick fix to their problem. Originally, the control group were scheduled to receive lifestyle changes for six months, but it was evident within three months that the subjects in this arm of the trial were not improving. They were therefore offered pelvic floor muscle exercises at the three-month assessment.

Five (9 per cent) subjects withdrew from the randomised controlled trial at three months. Of these, two (3.6 per cent) had regained normal function, making a total of three subjects (5.5 per cent) who dropped out without regaining normal function. This was less than in Van Kampen et al.'s (1998) (17.6 per cent), Claes et al.'s (1996b) (6.7 per cent) and Claes et al.'s (1995) (11.4 per cent) trials. In a trial using sildenafil for the treatment of erectile dysfunction in men with diabetes, Rendell et al. (1999) projected a patient dropout rate of 25 per cent. Similarly, in a trial using sildenafil for men with erectile dysfunction following radical prostatectomy, 21.4 per cent failed to complete follow-up IIEF questionnaires at eight weeks (Lowentritt et al., 1999). It was possible that more rigorous sample inclusion criteria, such as those used by Claes and Baert (1993), Claes et al. (1995) and Claes et al. (1996b), who included subjects with proven venous leakage, could have avoided some of the failures. Also, men were expected to attend for the digital anal examination and anal manometry and complete two lengthy questionnaires, which was considerably more arduous than reporting the categorical outcome, 'cured', 'improved' or 'failed' –

something that could be relayed by telephone. Another reason for withdrawal may be the embarrassment and reticence of British men compared to the Belgian men in Claes et al.'s trials. One subject aged 22 dropped out due to his aversion to the anal probe, which may have been particularly embarrassing in a man of his age.

Comparison with other trials

The majority of literature exploring the efficacy of pelvic floor muscle exercises for erectile dysfunction lacked randomisation and control groups, which limited the interpretation of findings. However, a number of factors were compared. These included the age of the subjects, the duration of erectile dysfunction and the severity of erectile dysfunction at baseline.

In this trial the median age of the subjects was 59.2 years – higher than the subjects in all the other trials, whose reported median ages were 53.3 years (Claes et al., 1996b), 49.5 years (Claes et al. (1995), 48.9 years (Claes and Baert, 1993), 39 years (Colpi et al., 1994) and 41.8 years (Lavoisier et al., 1986) respectively. In this trial, the Erectile Function domain of the IIEF was not correlated with the age of the subjects at baseline. However, it was found to correlate negatively with age in the intervention group at three months and the control group at six months after the pelvic floor muscle exercise regime. From this, it was possible to predict that younger men would benefit more from pelvic floor muscle exercises than older men. MacDonagh et al. (2002) reported that erectile dysfunction was viewed as a stigmatising condition and one that might lead to ridicule. They found that younger men found it easier than older men to discuss the condition with their partners. Older men were more likely to have relationship and communication difficulties. Age has been shown to be a risk factor for erectile dysfunction and usually means an increasing risk of developing other co-morbidities. These include hypertension, diabetes and heart disease, which may also affect erectile function (Wagner et al., 1996). Conversely, Van Kampen et al. (1998), who reported a mean age of 46 years (range 25–64 years), and Colpi et al. (1994) who reported a mean age of 39 years (range 20–63 years), concluded that age was not a determining factor for the success of pelvic floor muscle exercises.

The duration of erectile dysfunction was unreported in the majority of trials, but might have had implications for the comparison with this trial. Only Van Kampen et al. (1998) reported the mean duration of erectile dysfunction to be 46 months (range 2 months–30 years). The inclusion of a subject with a duration of only two months is questionable, as Cappelleri and Rosen (1999) considered that the diagnosis of erectile dysfunction should not be made until after at least six months' duration. In the current trial, all subjects had experienced erectile dysfunction for at least six months. At baseline, the mean duration was 72.4 months (range 6 months to 30 years), which was comparable in duration to the subjects in the trial by Van Kampen et al. (1998). In the current trial, three men who had experienced erectile dysfunction for 30 years failed to regain normal function. However, Van Kampen et al. (1998) reported that the duration of erectile dysfunction was not a predictor of the results of therapy, which was confirmed by the overall results of the current trial.

The severity of erectile dysfunction at baseline may have varied in the trials reviewed. In trials using sildenafil for subjects with mixed aetiology, baseline Erectile Function domain of the IIEF scores ranged between 10.4 and 13.5 points (Dinsmore et al., 1999; Tan et al., 2000). This indicated that subjects were less severe than in the current trial whose subjects' mean score at baseline was 9.15 points. This may have been due to a more rigorous screening process in the drug trials. Some of the trials using pelvic floor muscle exercises did not state the severity at baseline. Furthermore, the definition of erectile dysfunction may have differed. Claes et al. (1995) ranked subjects 'severe', 'moderate' or 'mild' according to pharmacological evaluation and Rigiscan, and found that improvements in penile rigidity from the 'mild' and 'moderate' group was significantly better than in the 'severe' group, whose results were all poor. In the current trial at baseline, 24 (43.6 per cent) subjects had a score of 0–6 ranked 'severe' in erectile function domain of the IIEF, and fourteen subjects (25.5 per cent) ranked 'moderate–severe' in the erectile function domain of the IIEF (see Table 2.5, p. 35). In the current trial, the severity of erectile dysfunction at baseline correlated with erectile function after intervention and home exercises in the control group, but failed to correlate with erectile function in the intervention group. This showed that the severity of erectile dysfunction at baseline was not found to be a risk factor in predicting a poor final outcome.

In comparison with a large grade II trial, pelvic floor muscle exercises were only slightly less effective than sildenafil in the same time frame (Goldstein et al., 1998) (see Table 5.7, p. 64). Interestingly, the improvement in the control arm of the Goldstein et al.'s (1998) study showed a placebo 'treatment effect' of two points on the Erectile Function Domain of the IIEF, in contrast to an improvement of only 0.6 points for the controls in the current trial (see Table 5.2 above). This may be explained by a psychological 'expectation effect' if the men believed they had received sildenafil. One could argue that the arm receiving sildenafil also improved slightly by the same psychological process. This favourable comparison with sildenafil further indicated that pelvic floor muscle exercises have merit as a realistic treatment for erectile dysfunction.

Analysis of the intervention

In the literature review, pelvic floor muscle exercises targeted at the ischiocavernosus and bulbocavernosus muscles appeared to have considerable merit as a treatment for erectile dysfunction for patients with venous leakage. They could also be useful for erectile dysfunction due to other causes such as poor musculature or a psychogenic origin. They were found to be non-invasive, easy to perform and free from side-effects.

In the current trial, pelvic floor muscle exercises were found to improve erectile dysfunction and post-micturition dribble significantly. The treatment regime focused on the ability to achieve maximum muscle contractions sustained for ten seconds, some sub-maximum contractions while walking and a strong post-void muscle contraction after micturition. No paper mentioned the supportive role of pelvic floor muscles. In order to achieve full fitness, maximal muscle work should be practised for muscle hypertrophy together with submaximal contractions for endurance (Guyton, 1986). Men can rehabilitate pelvic floor muscles for endurance by tightening and lifting up their pelvic floor about 50 per cent while walking and gradually increasing the time of the supportive lift. It is not necessary to perform pelvic floor muscle exercises with an erect penis following injection with papaverine as reported in Schouman and Lacroix (1991) and Claes and Baert (1993).

In normal men there is reflex activity in the pelvic floor muscles in response to functional demand. There may be an analogy between the loss of the rhabdosphincter reflex and the loss of urethrocavernosus and bulbocavernosus reflexes. The rhabdosphincter tightens in normal men by reflex action to prevent urine loss during increases in intra-abdominal pressure. This function can be relearned by using 'the knack' of voluntarily tightening the pelvic floor muscles during activities, which raise intra-abdominal pressure (Miller et al., 1996). Similarly, in the absence of reflex activity of the bulbocavernosus muscle, men can be taught to perform a voluntary 'squeeze-out' pelvic floor muscle contraction to eject the last few drops of urine after voiding. Strasser et al. (2001), using transrectal ultrasound after transurethral resection of prostate or radical prostatectomy, detected defects in the rhabdosphincter and post-operative scarring in seven out of twelve patients with post-operative stress incontinence. Of these, three patients showed areas of muscle thinning and two had complete rhabdosphincter atrophy. It may be that lack of use, benign prostatic hyperplasia or surgical intervention caused a level of atrophy of the bulbocavernosus muscle. It would be interesting to investigate the integrity of the bulbocavernosus muscle with these new imaging techniques. Voluntary muscle strengthening may not only serve to strengthen the bulbocavernosus muscle, but cortical control may have an influence on the autonomic system. It is not known whether these reflexes can be regained.

None of the trials agreed on the number of pelvic floor muscle contractions advised for daily home practice. Chang et al. (1998) instructed patients to perform 30 pelvic floor exercises 3–4 times a day, making a total of 90–120 exercises, while Porru et al. (2001) suggested 45 contractions a day. No trials have been performed on the minimum number of repetitions necessary. The principles of strength training demand maximum intensity rather than frequency. In other words, it is the quality of the muscle contraction not the quantity that is important. Muscle training depends on the motivation of the patient and adherence to the individual pelvic floor exercise regimen (Jackson et al., 1996). Men who are given an excessive number of exercises may well drop out from treatment.

The length of time for a muscle to achieve optimum strength depends on the initial muscle strength and the intensity of effort during training. Paterson et al. (1997) found that pelvic floor muscle tone took five weeks to build up to achieve a reduction in post-micturition dribble, while Chang et al. (1998) found that it took four weeks of pelvic floor muscle exercises before there was a significant reduction in post-micturition dribble.

Chang et al. (1998) instructed patients to interrupt the urinary stream with pelvic floor muscle exercises. It is thought inadvisable to teach mid-stream stopping as it reinforces the helplessness of those unable to stop the flow and counteracts the normal micturition reflexes by mimicking vesicosphincter dyssynergia (Bump et al., 1991). More seriously, it has been suggested that it produces a positive urethral closure pressure before the detrusor muscle contraction is suppressed, which can lead to reflux and eventually upper urinary tract injury (Bump et al., 1991).

It was impossible to determine from the literature or from the main trial whether biofeedback enhanced exercise performance or improved the effect of pelvic floor muscle exercises. During the intervention arm of the current trial, subjects practised their home exercises knowing they would be monitored with biofeedback at the five weekly sessions and at the assessment dates. Biofeedback provided motivation and encouragement to improve performance. Subjects strove to achieve a maximum contraction and to hold the contraction for ten seconds. Initially, thirteen (46.4 per cent) subjects in the intervention group and fifteen (55.6 per cent) in the control group (50.9 per cent of total sample) could hold the contraction for only 2–8 seconds, but following three months' pelvic floor muscle exercises, all subjects were able to maintain a ten-second hold. Clinicians conducting further trials may find biofeedback a useful method for enhancing performance.

Analysis of lifestyle changes

In the control group, no subject regained normal function following three months of advice on lifestyle changes. However, five (18.5 per cent) subjects reported improved rigidity, one (3.7 per cent) reported improved duration, seventeen (63.0 per cent) reported no improvement and one (3.7 per cent) reported worsening erectile dysfunction. It was expected that the control group would show some improvement by reducing alcohol levels, quitting smoking, increasing fitness levels, losing weight and avoiding saddle pressure. This did not seem to be the case. Although the majority of subjects reduced alcohol intake, lost some weight and performed daily exercises such as hill walking and running up and down stairs, no subject stopped smoking and two remained addicted to alcohol. As a group, the controls failed to improve during the three months of lifestyle changes. This was surprising. It was expected that subjects with a psychogenic cause to their erectile dysfunction would show improvement with lifestyle changes, and most patients do have a psychogenic component (Stief, 2002). It may be that three months of lifestyle changes was too short a time to effect a reversal of symptoms. However, after three months with no response the subjects were pleased to be offered pelvic floor muscle exercises.

This gave further strength to the finding that pelvic floor muscle exercises, and not psychological factors, caused the improvement in the intervention group. Erection confidence was significantly improved in the intervention group at three months ($p = 0.011$) compared to the control group ($p = 0.782$), and there was no significant improvement in the control group in the Erectile Function domain of the IIEF ($p = 0.658$) or any other category of the IIEF (see Table 5.4 above).

There may have been an effect from lifestyle changes over time. Following three months of lifestyle changes and three months of intervention, the control group increased the mean Erectile Function domain score from a baseline score of 7.45 to 18.27, a score difference of 10.82 points (p = 0.005) (see Table 5.7 above). The intervention group who received three months of intervention and lifestyle changes but no prior lifestyle advice increased the mean Erectile Function domain baseline score from 11.16 to 17.24, a score difference of 6.08 (p = 0.008) (see Table 5.6, p. 70). The greater improvement in the control group may have been due to increased adherence to the treatment regime. They may have benefited from encouragement from the therapist over a greater length of time, which may have increased motivation to comply with the home exercises and advice concerning lifestyle changes. The lifestyle changes may take longer to cause a beneficial effect and the controls may have shown a benefit at six months from the lifestyle advice received prior to the intervention.

Analysis of other factors

Selection of subjects

The selection criteria used in this trial closely matched the sort of men found in actual practice and is probably more representative than trials which have strict inclusion and exclusion criteria. In this trial, and in line with current treatment programmes, the subjects were not initially investigated with colour Doppler, intracavernous pharmacological evaluation, Rigiscan or nocturnal penile tumescence assessment. The cornerstone of clinical assessment remains a detailed sexual, medical and psychological history with identification of patient and partner needs (Wagner et al. (2002). Other trials have included subjects with proven venous leakage only (Mamberti-Dias and Bonierbale-Branchereau, 1991; Schouman and Lacroix, 1991; Claes and Baert, 1993; Colpi et al., 1994; Claes et al., 1995; Claes et al., 1996b). Only Van Kampen et al. (1998) included subjects with erectile dysfunction from a similar variety of causes. They monitored the causes of erectile dysfunction and found that the one significant factor related to outcome was the presence of veno-occlusive dysfunction (p = 0.0012). As the activity of the ischiocavernosus and bulbocavernosus muscles contribute to an increase in intracavernous pressure by compressing the deep dorsal vein of the penis, it seems reasonable to suppose that men with venous leakage due to weak pelvic floor musculature would benefit from strengthening exercises. From the results of the current trial for men of mixed aetiology, it has been possible to identify the criteria that might be applied in the future to evaluate more fully pelvic floor muscle exercises and manometric biofeedback for erectile dysfunction.

Study protocol

The study protocol was changed during the trial. It became clear that the control group would drop out if they continued to receive lifestyle changes only for six months as originally planned. Therefore, after three months they were offered the opportunity to cross over and receive the intervention and all patients in the control group agreed to receive pelvic floor muscle exercises at the three-month assessment.

Recruitment became a problem during the trial, so the change of protocol from a randomised controlled trial to a randomised cross-over parallel arm trial provided another sample of subjects to analyse. Also, due to problems of recruitment, a letter was sent to GPs requesting additional referrals to the trial.

Reasons for failures

Many subjects who failed to regain normal function were suffering from concomitant cardiovascular problems. Two had undergone cardiac bypass surgery, one suffered from cardiovascular problems and one had a pacemaker. In retrospect, it may have been better to have excluded men who may well have had an arteriogenic cause to their erectile dysfunction. Four of the men suffered from diabetes mellitus and may well have had early arteriosclerosis. These men were able to contract their pelvic floor muscles, so neurological impairment was ruled out. One subject had experienced erectile dysfunction for 30 years since undergoing bilateral orchidectomies and even with testosterone implants, failed to respond. One subject, who had Peyronie's disease, found penetration difficult and was referred for surgery. He may well have benefited from pelvic floor muscle exercises after surgery.

Two subjects complained of pain. One had experienced post-vasectomy testicular pain for 30 years; the other suffered discomfort from prostatitis. Shafik and El-Sibai (2000b) found pain from an anal fissure to be an inhibitor of sexual function. Similarly, it is possible that testicular or prostatic pain inhibits sexual function. One subject experienced low back pain while performing pelvic floor muscle exercises. He was the only subject who reported pain while exercising and was advised to find a comfortable position in which to practise his exercises. He was unable to find a pain-free position and may well find pelvic floor muscle exercises effective once his back symptoms have been successfully treated. Conversely, one subject who had suffered from proctalgia for three years reported that pelvic floor muscle exercises had relieved his prostatic pain and cured the seepage of semen he had previously experienced.

A high alcohol intake has been known to impair erectile function (Fabra and Porst, 1999). Two men had a daily intake of alcohol in excess of twelve units. Both reported a reduction of alcohol intake, but nevertheless arrived for treatment with alcohol on their breath. It may be that further trials should eliminate patients who consume high levels of alcohol as they are unlikely to benefit from treatment.

One subject had spent sixteen years bicycle racing and may have had a degree of saddle trauma. He was able to perform pelvic floor muscle exercises, which eliminated the possibility of paralysis of the pelvic floor muscles from pudendal nerve compression (Amarenco et al., 1987). However, perineal pressure has been found to compress the perineal arteries and decrease penile oxygen (Schwarzer et al., 2002). This may have been a possible aetiological factor in this case. Schwarzer et al. (2002) recommend a wide saddle which fully supports the pelvic bones and avoids perineal artery compression, but in this case, after such a long period, the damage may have been irreversible.

Three men were found to have low testosterone levels. They may well have benefited from testosterone replacement therapy prior to the trial. This might have had the effect of raising libido levels and interest in sexual activity. However, one could not be prescribed testosterone, as he was prone to anger following a head injury.

These co-morbidities provided a strong reason for future trials to be more selective and have a stricter exclusion criteria, which will exclude men with severe arteriogenic causes of erectile dysfunction, those with diabetes mellitus, men with a high intake of alcohol and men with low libido. However, few men have erectile dysfunction without other co-morbidities, which is a factor which has made the current trial more realistic than one performed under strict academic criteria.

Limitations of the study

The study was limited by the number of subjects. However, even with this limitation, it would appear that subjects with concomitant arteriogenic conditions and diabetes are unlikely to benefit from pelvic floor muscle exercises and should be excluded from further trials. Further trials could be multi-centred and thereby involve a larger sample size.

Another perceived limitation was the use of the unvalidated PIIEF. However, the inclusion of the PIIEF did involve partners in the research process and provided reinforcement to the accuracy of the subjects' IIEF responses. Results showed that 47 (85.5 per cent) partners were willing to take part. This indicated a need for a partner's questionnaire to be designed and validated, which would explain the problem from the partner's point of view and convey their own sexual and non-sexual needs in the relationship. It is possible that partners preferred forms of sexual activity other than vaginal penetration, which could be addressed and communicated to their men. The partner's IIEF also failed to address same-sex partners. Although all the men in this trial stated they were heterosexual, a partner's questionnaire is needed that addresses the needs and wishes of same-sex partners.

The trial was also limited by the lack of a blind assessment at baseline and by the blind assessor having knowledge of the trial hypothesis. Either factor could have led to bias. However, the blind assessment was not the main outcome measure, but added support to outcomes from the IIEF and anal manometry to provide triangulation of data.

Analysis of outcome measures for post-micturition dribble

At baseline, none of the subjects reported any form of incontinence other than post-micturition dribble, which affected 21 subjects in the intervention group and fifteen in the control group. Unfortunately, the outcome measures were subjective due to the failure of the pad tests to weigh small amounts of leakage. However, blind assessors were used to avoid bias. Post-micturition dribble was assessed by the single question: 'Did you suffer from post-micturition dribble? If so is it now Worse, Same, Less amount of leakage, Less amount of leakage and less often, or Cured?' The large percentage of subjects that were cured (75 per cent) strengthened the argument that pelvic floor muscle exercises and the post-void 'squeeze-out' muscle contraction were realistic treatments for post-micturition dribble in men. Interestingly, all subjects suffering from post-micturition dribble at baseline reported to the clinician following intervention that they were able to squeeze out some more drops of urine during the 'squeeze-out' muscle contraction. Subsequently, all subjects experienced no further dribbling. This ability to squeeze out a few more drops may have been conveyed to the blind assessor as 'after-dribble' and therefore skewed the results. The clinician asked 'After you have tightened your muscles and "squeezed out" a few more drops over the toilet, do you have any further leakage of urine when you leave the bathroom?', whereas the blind assessor asked 'Did you suffer from post-micturition dribble before the trial? How is it now?' This shows the importance of clear and unambiguous questioning in order to gain a true treatment outcome. Further trials are needed to confirm these self-reported findings.

Association between erectile dysfunction and post-micturition dribble

The results suggest that there may be an association between erectile dysfunction and post-micturition dribble. This was the first time that an association between the two has been specifically explored. In the randomised controlled part of this trial using a sample of 55 subjects with erectile dysfunction, pelvic floor muscle exercises were found to be significantly effective after three months to improve erectile function ($p = 0.001$). Overall, after three months of pelvic floor muscle exercises and three months of home exercises, 22 (40 per cent) men regained normal erectile function, nineteen (34.5 per cent) improved and fourteen (25.5 per cent) dropped out or failed to improve. At baseline, it was found that 36 (65.5 per cent) subjects also suffered from post-micturition dribble. Following the regime of pelvic floor muscle exercises, 27 (75 per cent) subjects were cured, three (8.3 per cent) improved, five (13.9 per cent) dropped out and one (2.8 per cent) failed to improve. The literature review on pelvic floor muscle exercises for erectile dysfunction found that pelvic floor muscle training could improve the outcome of men suffering from erectile dysfunction due to venous leakage. The literature review on pelvic floor muscle exercises for post-micturition dribble found that the bulbocavernosus reflex emptied the bulbar portion of the urethra in normal men and that pelvic floor muscle exercises could cure or improve post-micturition dribble. This current grade II level of evidence trial has added to previous knowledge and has supported the idea that pelvic floor muscle dysfunction may have a causal link associated with both conditions. This combined evidence adds strength to the argument that there is an association between the conditions of erectile dysfunction and post-micturition dribble due to dysfunction of the pelvic floor musculature.

Chapter 8
Implications of the study

Contribution to knowledge

The results of this randomised controlled cross-over parallel arm trial adds to the current body of knowledge in two main areas. Evidence has shown that pelvic floor muscle exercises are significantly effective for some men with erectile dysfunction. Evidence has also shown that the same exercises are significantly effective in the treatment of men with post-micturition dribble. The current trial showed that a post-void 'squeeze-out' muscle contraction was effective for post-micturition dribble. To obtain a benefit, pelvic floor muscle exercises should be taught and practised for up to six months. A maintenance programme may then be implemented for life.

Anal manometric measurements have been shown to be a reliable outcome measure for men with erectile difficulties. These measurements correlated well with digital anal measurements, but there is a need for reassessment of the digital anal grade in men.

Who will benefit?

The results show that men with weak pelvic floor muscles and men with a venogenic cause of erectile dysfunction benefit by strengthening the ischiocavernosus and bulbocavernosus muscles together with the pelvic floor musculature. Men with a psychological cause may also benefit. Linear regression analysis has shown that younger men performing pelvic floor muscle exercises may have a better chance of regaining erectile function than older men.

Who will not benefit?

Not all men with erectile dysfunction are suitable for pelvic floor muscle training. Men with a severe arteriogenic cause, such as cardio-vascular disease and arteriosclerosis, and men taking anti-hypertensive medication may not benefit. Also, men with congenital abnormalities, diabetes mellitus and neurological conditions may not derive benefit. Men with a high alcohol intake may not improve. Those men with a low libido would be advised to receive testosterone replacement prior to treatment, and men with severe Peyronie's disease would be advised to undergo surgery before commencing treatment. It is also advisable for men with severe back or pelvic pain to receive pain-relief before embarking on a course of pelvic floor muscle exercises.

Management pathways for erectile dysfunction

Pelvic floor muscle exercises can be considered as a first-line approach for men seeking long-term resolution of erectile dysfunction without acute pharmacological and surgical interventions that may have more significant side-effects. Men demanding a 'quick fix' may prefer to restore normal muscle function once they understand the important role of the pelvic floor muscles. Following routine muscle testing at prostate and erectile dysfunction clinics, men with weak pelvic floor muscles may be more amenable to this regime. Also, men receiving other forms of therapy for erectile dysfunction could be advised to prac-tise pelvic floor muscle exercises in addition to the therapy prescribed.

A suggested management pathway for men with erectile dysfunction is shown (Figure 8.1).

How the results will change practice

The results of this research will change practice in a number of ways. Some changes will be instigated by professionals and some will be patient-driven. Specialist continence physiotherapists and continence specialist nurses working at this level base current practice on the avail-able evidence. This research provides more evidence on which to base clinical practice. Urology assessments by all medical practitioners, including nurses and physiotherapists, could include a single question 'Do you have difficulty attaining or maintaining an erection?', which would present an opportunity to offer pelvic floor muscle exercises. Pelvic floor muscles could be graded digitally at urology examinations, such as at prostate clinics, and those men with weak pelvic floor

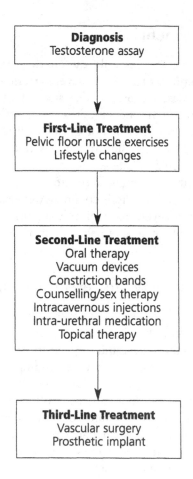

Figure 8.1: Suggested algorithm for treatment of erectile dysfunction

musculature could be offered a strengthening regime. It also seems reasonable to suggest preventative exercises. Many men never consciously work their pelvic floor muscles. Men with sedentary occupations and hobbies may be well advised to exercise their pelvic floor muscles during periods of inactivity. Men undergoing prostate or abdominal surgery could strengthen their muscles before and after surgery. Workouts in the gym could include exercises for the pelvic floor in order to develop all muscles equally and avoid muscle imbalance. Also, professionals could ask if their patients are bothered by post-micturition dribble. Men who experience this condition could then be given an appropriate pelvic floor muscle exercise regime and taught the 'squeeze-out' muscle contraction.

The role of the patient is changing. The public is gaining an increasing amount of medical knowledge through a range of media including the internet, and the concept of the 'Expert Patient' is evolving by those who take an active role in their care (Department of Health, 2001). These patients are questioning cure rates, side-effects and risks of all treatment modalities. Professionals can provide that evidence and prescribe conservative therapies such as pelvic floor muscle exercises as a first-line approach before other, more invasive regimes, are implemented. Disturbingly, a questionnaire sent to 300 GPs in England found that only 2 per cent used physiotherapy as their first choice for soft tissue injury due to access difficulties and extended waiting lists, even though 93 per cent rated physiotherapy as effective or very effective (Carter et al., 2001). By promoting their role and clinical effectiveness, physiotherapists may increase the rate of referrals, but resource issues have to be addressed.

Chapter 9
Dissemination of results

Advancement of physiotherapy

Introduction

'Advanced practice in physiotherapy' is termed as a level of skill that reaches beyond mainstream practice, with Chartered Society of Physiotherapy members identifying their own standard of practice at advanced level (Chartered Society of Physiotherapy, 1995). In the UK, Stewart (1998) considered advanced practice in physiotherapy to be at the cutting edge of professional advancement. This model recognised that physiotherapists may not be carrying out physiotherapy as defined by the Chartered Society of Physiotherapy and may be experts in a recognised field other than physiotherapy. It considered that physiotherapists may be expanding and developing the profession by involvement in research, education and management. It valued the contribution of lecturers from academia who can contribute to the body of knowledge of recognised physiotherapy practice. The model considered that advanced practice was dynamic, with its evolution informed by research. It should bring about improved change in practice and assumed that advanced practice would lead to better patient outcomes in line with the changing NHS. Advanced practice in this model includes the dissemination of knowledge to peers and others as a regular feature of practice.

The profile of physiotherapy has never been higher and physiotherapists are now recognised as innovators and leaders capable of effecting change at every level (Chadda, 2002). The role of good, evidence-based research is deemed pivotal to the development of the advanced practitioner (Stewart, 1998).

Clinicians have an important role to play in developing a specific knowledge base and undertaking sound research to maximise the quality of clinical practice, whereas academics have certain advantages working in a research-oriented institution (Helders et al., 1999).

Richardson (1993) argues that, unlike in the past, research should be driven by practice rather than by academic interest, thereby helping to narrow the gap between theory and practice.

Contribution to the advancement of physiotherapy

The combination of a specialist clinical role with that of a PhD student has provided the physiotherapy profession with the first grade II level of evidence study in a novel specialist area. The extensive literature reviews and the critical thinking in this volume have further confirmed the merit of pelvic floor muscle exercises for erectile dysfunction. This is the first time that erectile dysfunction has been associated with post-micturition dribble due to weak musculature affecting both erectile function and the normal post-void bulbocavernosus muscle function.

This research should generate a change in physiotherapy practice. The author in her role as a clinical specialist is currently having men with erectile dysfunction referred to her for treatment with pelvic floor muscle exercises by the local erectile dysfunction clinic. These men are receiving 2–5 treatments of pelvic floor muscle exercise. For practice to change, it will be necessary to provide specific education for the professionals in the specialty, general education for health professionals not in the specialty and clear literature for the public. It is most likely that change will initially be managed by urologists, nurses working in erectile dysfunction clinics and by physiotherapists and nurses working in the field of continence.

Role of consultant physiotherapist in continence

The term 'continence' is used in this specialty in preference to the negative term 'incontinence'. Recent reforms have created opportunities for physiotherapy services to develop extended scope practitioner and consultant posts at advanced practitioner grades (Chartered Society of Physiotherapy, 2001). Former Health Secretary Alan Milburn expressed a wish to have 250 consultant therapists in post by 2005 (Byrne, 2002). In the field of continence, there is a unique opportunity for physiotherapists to work as 'consultant physiotherapists in continence'. Applicants would probably need experience at PhD level and proven clinical specialist skill. Successful candidates could enhance the service in a number of key directions. They could develop and manage a conservative continence service for men and women with clear guidelines and defined protocols. They could receive direct referrals and work as a first-line conservative continence practitioner, with the ability to request investigations, such as urine analysis and flow tests, and with open referral access to other members of the multi-disciplinary team. They could have responsibility for training physiotherapists and nurses at all levels in the hospital and in the community and also undertake the evaluation of practice and the audit of the service. In this role, they would have the ability to design and conduct much needed research at a high level in the clinical setting and within the local community. Service users, providers and educators are increasingly aware of the need for highly skilled health professionals who can respond to, and influence, changes to practice and service delivery (Donaghy and Gosling, 1999). Conversely, Durrell (1996) highlights the implicit risk of deskilling the physiotherapy department by removing its clinical specialists. However, it can be argued that these new roles would help retain clinical specialists in a dual role with benefits to both the physiotherapy and urology departments. This novel post would present a unique opportunity for career progression, advanced level practice and further good quality research. It would also provide a forum for the dissemination of the results of this research.

Dissemination of results

The results of this research will be disseminated to professionals and to the public. Physiotherapy educators are in a position to make a contribution to the development of both the profession of physiotherapy and to education (Morris, 2002).

Dissemination to professionals

The results of this research will be disseminated to urologists specialising in sexual dysfunction, general practitioners, nurses working in continence and erectile dysfunction clinics and physiotherapists specialising in male continence. In order to reach those medical professionals who have the ability to change practice, groups will be targeted through relevant medical peer-reviewed journals. Another way to target urologists, physiotherapists and nurses is by lecturing at international and national conferences.

Dissemination to the public

Dissemination to the public could take the form of lectures, leaflets and patient booklets. Lectures could be offered to groups, such as those over 50 years of age in the Rotary Club. It may be prudent to offer lectures to under-50s too. As some of the partners instigated the referral process, lectures could be offered to women's clubs, or it may be that a mixed audience would be receptive. The author would include the results of this research in the next edition of the patient book *Use it or Lose it!* (Dorey, 2001d), but to reach the general public a low-cost leaflet has been produced for availability in public areas, such as GP surgeries, health clinics and hospital waiting areas.

Recommendations for further research

Pelvic floor muscle exercises for erectile dysfunction

Further investigation is required to ascertain which categories of men will benefit most from pelvic floor muscle exercises. A large, multi-centre, cross-cultural randomised controlled study could be designed to provide insight into the sub-groups likely to benefit from pelvic floor muscle exercises. It would be interesting to ascertain whether the results of this trial could be replicated by others, in different settings, with a heterogeneous sample of men with erectile dysfunction.

The sample size should include a minimum of 37 subjects in each group. This power calculation is based on the data from the current trial giving a between-group score difference of 5.3 points in the Erectile Function domain of the IIEF at three months with a standard deviation of 8. It would detect a difference of 5.3 points at the 5 per cent significance level with 80 per cent power.

$$n = \frac{SD^2}{SE^2}$$

n = sample size
SD = standard deviation
SE = standard error

Further investigation is required into the use of pelvic floor muscle exercises in a preventive role, to avoid or delay the onset of erectile dysfunction. A long-term randomised controlled multi-centre cross-cultural study could be designed to explore the effects of pelvic floor exercise in normal men, in order to ascertain their use as a preventative measure for erectile dysfunction. The sample could include men of all ages with normal erectile function.

It is still not known whether fewer good quality contractions are preferable to exercising many times a day. It may be that vigorous exercise is necessary only three times a week. Therefore, a randomised controlled study could be designed to explore the number of pelvic floor muscle exercises that should be performed to improve erectile dysfunction. This could involve annual follow-up assessments as the compliance of men practising pelvic floor muscle exercises long-term remains unknown.

Further work needs to be done on the role of manometric biofeed-back. A randomised controlled study could be designed to ascertain whether biofeedback enhances pelvic floor muscle exercises.

Pelvic floor muscle exercises for post-micturition dribble

Further investigation is required to ascertain which categories of men will benefit from pelvic floor muscle exercises and a post-void 'squeeze-out' muscle contraction for post-micturition dribble. A large, multi-centre cross-cultural randomised controlled study could be designed to provide additional insight into the sub-groups of men who could be offered this treatment.

Another long-term randomised controlled study could be designed to explore the effects of pelvic floor muscle exercises and a post-void 'squeeze-out' muscle contraction for normal men of all ages in order to ascertain their use as a preventive measure for post-micturition dribble.

Outcome measures

Partner's quality of life questionnaire

Further work needs to be done to produce a valid, reliable and sensitive outcome measure to assess the impact of erectile dysfunction on the quality of life and social activities of partners. Validation of such a questionnaire should include input from partners of different sexes, sexual preferences, ages, cultures, and religions.

Anal pressure measurements

Further investigation of the reliability of anal pressure measurements is required. This includes the assessment of inter-rater reliability and a more detailed analysis of within-day reliability to assess the minimal number of measurements required to obtain clinically reliable results for this invasive procedure. A further study could use the same men for both within-day and day-to-day analysis of reliability, thus allowing direct comparison of results.

More work needs to be done to investigate the correlation of anal manometry with digital anal examination and also anal EMG. This study could reassess the digital anal grades in men.

Further research conclusion

These suggestions would build on the current study, which has reached beyond mainstream practice and contributed to the growth of the profession by pushing the boundaries still further into the realms of 'Advanced practice in physiotherapy' in an innovative area.

Importantly, it has the potential to improve significantly the health of the public.

Conclusion

This randomised controlled cross-over parallel arm trial has offered evidence from a validated outcome measure that pelvic floor muscle exercises are effective therapies for a significant proportion of men with erectile dysfunction and for post-micturition dribble. It has established an association between both conditions due to pelvic floor muscle dysfunction. It has introduced the concept of a post-void 'squeeze-out' muscle contraction to eliminate post-micturition dribble.

Anal manometric measurements have been shown to be a reliable outcome measure for men with erectile difficulties. Anal manometric measurements were found to correlate well with digital anal measurements although the digital anal grades need to be reassessed in men.

The results of this trial will be disseminated to health professionals including urologists, GPs, nurses and physiotherapists. Steps will be taken to inform the public of the outcome of this research.

It is hoped to build on the extensive knowledge gained from this level II evidence research, and perform a multi-centred, cross-cultural study into pelvic floor muscle exercises for men with erectile difficulties. This will provide the specialty with level I evidence research on which to base practice.

Appendix 1

International Index of Erectile Function

Your answers will be strictly confidential and only used for research purposes.

These questions ask about the effects your erection problems have had on your sex life *over the past four weeks*. Please answer the following questions as honestly and clearly as possible. In answering these questions, the following definitions apply:

- **sexual activity**: includes intercourse, caressing, foreplay and masturbation
- **sexual intercourse**: is defined as vaginal penetration of the partner (you entered your partner)
- **sexual stimulation**: includes situations like foreplay with a partner, looking at pictures, etc.
- **ejaculate**: the ejection of semen from the penis (or the feeling of this)

1. *Over the past four weeks*, how often were you able to get an erection during sexual activity?

Please tick one box only
[0] No sexual activity
[5] Almost always or always
[4] Most times (much more than half the time)
[3] Sometimes (about half the time)
[2] A few times (much less than half the time)
[1] Almost never or never

Please turn over

2. *Over the past four weeks*, when you had erections with sexual stimulation, how often were your erections hard enough for penetration?

Please tick one box only
[0]   No sexual stimulation
[5]   Almost always or always
[4]   Most times (much more than half the time)
[3]   Sometimes (about half the time)
[2]   A few times (much less than half the time)
[1]   Almost never or never

The next three questions will ask about the erections you may have had during sexual intercourse.

3. *Over the past four weeks*, when you attempted sexual intercourse, how often were you able to penetrate (enter) your partner?

Please tick one box only
[0]   Did not attempt intercourse
[5]   Almost always or always
[4]   Most times (much more than half the time)
[3]   Sometimes (about half the time)
[2]   A few times (much less than half the time)
[1]   Almost never or never

4. *Over the past four weeks*, during sexual intercourse, *how often:* were you able to maintain your erection after you had penetrated (entered) your partner?

Please tick one box only
[0]   Did not attempt intercourse
[5]   Almost always or always
[4]   Most times (much more than half the time)
[3]   Sometimes (about half the time)
[2]   A few times (much less than half the time)
[1]   Almost never or never

5. *Over the past four weeks*, during sexual intercourse, *how difficult* was it to maintain your erection to completion of intercourse?

Please tick one box only
[0]   Did not attempt intercourse
[1]   Extremely difficult
[2]   Very difficult
[3]   Difficult
[4]   Slightly difficult
[5]   Not difficult

6. *Over the past four weeks*, how many times have you attempted sexual intercourse?

Please tick one box only
[0]   No attempts
[1]   1–2 attempts
[2]   3–4 attempts
[3]   5–6 attempts
[4]   7-10 attempts
[5]   11+ attempts

7. *Over the past four weeks*, when you attempted sexual intercourse, how *often* was it satisfactory for you?

Please tick one box only
[0]   Did not attempt intercourse
[5]   Almost always or always
[4]   Most times (much more than half the time)
[3]   Sometimes (about half the time)
[2]   A few times (much less than half the time)
[1]   Almost never or never

8. *Over the past four weeks*, how much have you enjoyed sexual intercourse?

Please tick one box only
[0]   No intercourse
[5]   Very highly enjoyable
[4]   Highly enjoyable
[3]   Fairly enjoyable
[2]   Not very enjoyable
[1]   No enjoyment

Please turn over

9. *Over the past four weeks*, when you had sexual stimulation or intercourse, how often did you ejaculate?

Please tick one box only
[0]   No sexual stimulation / intercourse
[5]   Almost always or always
[4]   Most times (much more than half the time)
[3]   Sometimes (about half the time)
[2]   A few times (much less than half the time)
[1]   Almost never or never

10. *Over the past four weeks*, when you had sexual stimulation or intercourse how often did you have a feeling of orgasm (with or without ejaculation?

Please tick one box only
[0]   No sexual stimulation/intercourse
[5]   Almost always or always
[4]   Most times (much more than half the time)
[3]   Sometimes (about half the time)
[2]   A few times (much less than half the time)
[1]   Almost never or never

The next two questions ask about sexual desire. Let's define sexual desire as a feeling that may include wanting to have a sexual experience (for example masturbation or intercourse), thinking about having sex, or feeling frustrated due to lack of sex.

11. *Over the past four weeks*, how often have you felt *sexual desire*?

Please tick one box only
[5]   Almost always or always
[4]   Most times (much more than half the time)
[2]   Sometimes (about half the time)
[3]   A few times (much less than half the time)
[1]   Almost never or never

12. *Over the past four weeks*, how would you rate your level of sexual desire?

Please tick one box only
[5]   Very high
[4]   High
[3]   Moderate
[2]   Low
[1]   Very low or none at all

13. *Over the past four weeks*, how satisfied have you been with your overall *sex life*?

Please tick one box only
[5]   Very satisfied
[4]   Moderately satisfied
[3]   About equally satisfied and dissatisfied
[2]   Moderately dissatisfied
[1]   Very dissatisfied

14. *Over the past four weeks*, how satisfied have you been with your sexual relationship with your partner?

Please tick one box only
[5]   Very satisfied
[4]   Moderately satisfied
[3]   About equally satisfied and dissatisfied
[2]   Moderately dissatisfied
[1]   Very dissatisfied

15. *Over the past four weeks*, how do you rate your *confidence* in getting and keeping an erection?

Please tick one box only
[5]   Very high
[4]   High
[3]   Moderate
[2]   Low
[1]   Very low

Thank you for completing this questionnaire.

Appendix 2
Erectile Dysfunction – Effect on Quality of Life Questionnaire

This questionnaire asks for your views about your erectile problem. Please read each item and place a tick in the box opposite the reply which comes closest to how you feel.

1. As a result of your erectile difficulties, do you blame yourself for being unable to satisfy your partner?

Not at all	A little	Somewhat	Quite a lot	A great deal
☐	☐	☐	☐	☐

2. Does your inability to produce an erection with your partner make you feel guilty?

Not at all	A little	Somewhat	Quite a lot	A great deal
☐	☐	☐	☐	☐

3. Do you feel less desirable as a result of your erectile difficulties?

Not at all	A little	Somewhat	Quite a lot	A great deal
☐	☐	☐	☐	☐

4. Do you feel hurt by your partner's response to your erectile difficulties?

Not at all	A little	Somewhat	Quite a lot	A great deal
☐	☐	☐	☐	☐

5. Does the fact that you are unable to produce an erection make you feel less of a man?

Not at all	A little	Somewhat	Quite a lot	A great deal
☐	☐	☐	☐	☐

6. Do you feel angry or bitter that you cannot produce an erection?

Not at all	A little	Somewhat	Quite a lot	A great deal
☐	☐	☐	☐	☐

7. Do you feel a failure because of your erectile difficulties?

Not at all	A little	Somewhat	Quite a lot	A great deal
☐	☐	☐	☐	☐

Please read each item and place a tick opposite the reply that comes closest to how you feel.

1. Does your partner feel let down by your inability to produce an erection?

Not at all	A little	Somewhat	Quite a lot	A great deal
☐	☐	☐	☐	☐

2. Are you worried that your erectile problems have affected the closeness between you and your partner?

Not at all	A little	Somewhat	Quite a lot	A great deal
☐	☐	☐	☐	☐

3. Does your erectile problem make you worry about how your life will develop in the future?

Not at all	A little	Somewhat	Quite a lot	A great deal
☐	☐	☐	☐	☐

4. Is your sense of identity altered by your lack of erectile function?

Not at all	A little	Somewhat	Quite a lot	A great deal
☐	☐	☐	☐	☐

5. Are you preoccupied by your erection problems?

Not at all	A little	Somewhat	Quite a lot	A great deal
☐	☐	☐	☐	☐

6. Do you feel sad or tearful as a result of your erectile difficulties?

Not at all	A little	Somewhat	Quite a lot	A great deal
☐	☐	☐	☐	☐

7. Do you feel that other people are happier than you are because they are sexually fulfilled?

Not at all	A little	Somewhat	Quite a lot	A great deal
☐	☐	☐	☐	☐

8. Is your self-esteem damaged by your erectile problems?

Not at all	A little	Somewhat	Quite a lot	A great deal
☐	☐	☐	☐	☐

Thank you for completing this questionnaire.

Taunton and Somerset NHS Trust, 1998.

Appendix 3
Partner's International Index of Erectile Function

Please fill this in *without* your partner's help. Your answers will be strictly confidential and only used for research purposes.

Please do not discuss your responses to this questionnaire with your partner. When you have completed this questionnaire please send it to Grace Dorey in the stamped addressed envelope provided.

These questions ask about the effects your partner's erection problems have had on his sex life *over the past four weeks*. Please answer the following questions as honestly and clearly as possible. In answering these questions, the following definitions apply:

- **sexual activity** includes intercourse, caressing, foreplay and masturbation
- **sexual intercourse** is defined as vaginal penetration by your partner
- **sexual stimulation** includes situations like foreplay with your partner, looking at pictures, etc.
- **ejaculate**: the ejection of semen from your partner's penis (or his feeling of this)

1. *Over the past four weeks*, how often has your partner been able to get an erection during sexual activity?

Please tick one box only
[0]   No sexual activity
[5]   Almost always or always
[4]   Most times (much more than half the time)
[3]   Sometimes (about half the time)
[2]   A few times (much less than half the time)
[1]   Almost never or never

2. *Over the past four weeks*, when your partner had erections with sexual stimulation, how often were his erections hard enough for penetration?

Please tick one box only
[0]   No sexual stimulation
[5]   Almost always or always
[4]   Most times (much more than half the time)
[3]   Sometimes (about half the time)
[2]   A few times (much less than half the time)
[1]   Almost never or never

The next three questions will ask about your partner's erections during sexual intercourse.

3. *Over the past four weeks*, when your partner attempted sexual intercourse, how often was your partner able to penetrate you?

Please tick one box only
[0]   Did not attempt intercourse
[5]   Almost always or always
[4]   Most times (much more than half the time)
[3]   Sometimes (about half the time)
[2]   A few times (much less than half the time)
[1]   Almost never or never

4. *Over the past four weeks*, during sexual intercourse, how often was your partner able to maintain his erection after he had penetrated (entered) you?

Please tick one box only
[0]   Did not attempt intercourse
[5]   Almost always or always
[4]   Most times (much more than half the time)
[3]   Sometimes (about half the time)
[2]   A few times (much less than half the time)
[1]   Almost never or never

Please turn over

5. *Over the past four weeks*, during sexual intercourse, how difficult was it for your partner to maintain his erection to completion of intercourse?

Please tick one box only
[0]   Did not attempt intercourse
[1]   Extremely difficult
[2]   Very difficult
[3]   Difficult
[4]   Slightly difficult
[5]   Not difficult

6. *Over the past four weeks*, how many times has your partner attempted sexual intercourse?

Please tick one box only
[0]   No attempts
[1]   1–2 attempts
[2]   3–4 attempts
[3]   5–6 attempts
[4]   7–10 attempts
[5]   11+ attempts

7. *Over the past four weeks*, when your partner attempted sexual intercourse, how often was it satisfactory for him?

Please tick one box only
[0]   Did not attempt intercourse
[5]   Almost always or always
[4]   Most times (much more than half the time)
[3]   Sometimes (about half the time)
[2]   A few times (much less than half the time)
[1]   Almost never or never

8. *Over the past four weeks*, how much has your partner enjoyed sexual intercourse?

Please tick one box only
[0]   No intercourse
[5]   Very highly enjoyable
[4]   Highly enjoyable
[3]   Fairly enjoyable
[2]   Not very enjoyable
[1]   No enjoyment

9. *Over the past four weeks*, when your partner had sexual stimulation or intercourse, how often did he ejaculate?

Please tick one box only
[0]   No sexual stimulation/intercourse
[5]   Almost always or always
[4]   Most times (much more than half the time)
[3]   Sometimes (about half the time)
[2]   A few times (much less than half the time)
[1]   Almost never or never

10. *Over the past four weeks*, when your partner had sexual stimulation or intercourse how often did he have a feeling of orgasm (with or without ejaculation)?

Please tick one box only
[0]   No sexual stimulation/intercourse
[5]   Almost always or always
[4]   Most times (much more than half the time)
[3]   Sometimes (about half the time)
[2]   A few times (much less than half the time)
[1]   Almost never or never

The next two questions ask about your partner's sexual desire. Let's define sexual desire as a feeling by your partner that may include wanting to have a sexual experience (for example, masturbation or intercourse), thinking about having sex, or feeling frustrated due to lack of sex.

11. *Over the past four weeks*, how often has your partner felt sexual desire?

Please tick one box only
[5]   Almost always or always
[4]   Most times (much more than half the time)
[3]   Sometimes (about half the time)
[2]   A few times (much less than half the time)
[1]   Almost never or never

Please turn over

12. *Over the past four weeks,* how would you rate your partner's level of sexual desire?

Please tick one box only
[5]   Very high
[4]   High
[3]   Moderate
[2]   Low
[1]   Very low or none at all

13. *Over the past four weeks,* how satisfied has your partner been with your overall sex life?

Please tick one box only
[5]   Very satisfied
[4]   Moderately satisfied
[3]   About equally satisfied and dissatisfied
[2]   Moderately dissatisfied
[1]   Very dissatisfied

14. *Over the past four weeks,* how satisfied has your partner been with your sexual relationship?

Please tick one box only
[5]   Very satisfied
[4]   Moderately satisfied
[3]   About equally satisfied and dissatisfied
[2]   Moderately dissatisfied
[1]   Very dissatisfied

15. *Over the past four weeks,* how do you rate your partner's confidence in getting and keeping an erection?

Please tick one box only
[5]   Very high
[4]   High
[3]   Moderate
[2]   Low
[1]   Very low

Thank you for completing this questionnaire.

When you have completed this questionnaire please send it in the stamped addressed envelope provided to:
Grace Dorey MSc MCSP
Physiotherapy Department
The Somerset Nuffield Hospital
Staplegrove Elm
Taunton
Somerset TA2 6AN

Male Continence Subjective Assessment Form

Patient details

Date
_____

Name
_____

Address
_____

Telephone no.
_____

Date of birth /Age
_____

Occupation
_____

Hobbies/activities
_____

Source of referral
_____

Consultant
_____

GP
_____

Problem

Main problem
_____

Length of time for main problem
_____

Mild   Moderate   Severe
_____

Limitation of activities
_____

Quality of life due to urinary problem
_____

Bothersome rating: 0 1 2 3 4 5 6 7 8 9 10

Symptoms

Stress
_____

Urgency
_____

Urge incontinence
_____

Provoking factors
_____

Awareness of leakage
_____
Frequency
_____
Nocturia
_____
Nocturnal enuresis
_____
Description of flow rate
_____
Poor sensation of micturition
_____
Hesitation starting to pass urine
_____
Difficulty passing urine
_____
Weak stream
_____
Small voids
_____
Terminal dribble
_____
Post-void dribble
_____
Constant dribble
_____
Does bladder feel full after voiding
_____
Dysuria
_____
Haematuria, dark or smoky urine
_____
Pain: suprapubic, genital, perineal, testes, penis (mark on body chart)
_____
Childhood urinary problems
_____

Severity of symptoms (Visual analogue scale 0–10 for each symptom)
Symptom 1   0 1 2 3 4 5 6 7 8 9 10
_____
Symptom 2   0 1 2 3 4 5 6 7 8 9 10
_____
Symptom 3   0 1 2 3 4 5 6 7 8 9 10

Duration of symptoms
Length of time for Symptom 1
_____
Length of time for Symptom 2
_____
Length of time for Symptom 3
_____
Improvement or deterioration to date
_____

Amount of leakage

Few drops	Spurt		Large leakage
No. of pads per day	Damp	Wet	Soaked
Type of appliance			
ISC			
Indwelling catheter Size	Number of days used		

Frequency of leakage
Daily >1 / week <1 / week >1 / month <1 / month
_____
Time of day leakage occurs
_____
Leakage aggravators: Coughing   Sneezing   Walking
Moving Running water   Caffeine   Alcohol
Medications   Other:
_____

Urine stop test (not to be used as an exercise)
Stop   Slow down   Unable to stop
_____

Bowel activity
Constipation
_____
Straining to defaecate
_____
Number of times defaecates per week
_____
Stool: Liquid   Soft   Firm
_____
Faecal urgency
_____
Faecal incontinence
_____
Incontinence of flatus
_____
Laxatives
_____
Diet
_____

Surgical history
TURP   Date   Outcome
_____
Radical prostatectomy   Date   Outcome
_____
Urethral stricture   Date
_____
Other surgery
_____

Medical history
Family history
_____
Prostatitis: Acute   Chronic   No. of episodes
_____
Cystitis: Acute   Chronic   No. of episodes
_____
Latex allergy
_____
Metal implants
_____
Heart problems
_____
Smoking
_____
Respiratory problems
_____
Other problems
_____

Anticholinergic medications:
Tolterodine (detrusitol) Oxybutynin (ditropan)

Alpha blockers (relax bladder neck)
Doxazosin mesylate (Cardura)

5 alpha reductase inhibitors (reduces size of prostate)
Finasteride (Proscar)

Anti-androgen drug treatment

Other medications

Effect of medication

Side-effects of medication

Radiotherapy

Neurological problems:
Diabetes   MS   Parkinson's   Other

Lumbar or cervical spine problems
with neurological deficit

Previous treatment
Previous physiotherapy and outcome

Body mass index
Height   metres

Weight   kg

BMI (weight in kg divided by height in metres squared:
BMI >30 = obese)

Sexual problems
Difficulty achieving erection

Difficulty maintaining erection

Inability to gain erection

Functional factors
Position used for urination

Mobility and dexterity

Environmental factors

Cognitive/mental abilities

Psychological state

Patient support system

Motivation
Ability to incorporate therapy into lifestyle

Investigations
Urinalysis of MSU
(essential)

Uroflow
(essential if physiotherapist is first contact)

Post-void residual
(essential if physiotherapist is first contact)

Ultrasound scan
(of interest)

Urodynamics including post void residual and uroflow
(helpful)

Flexible cystoscopy for diagnosis of stricture and tumours
(helpful)

Frequency/volume chart (home and work days; ideally seven days)
Frequency of voiding

Maximum voided volume

Minimum voided volume

Amount of fluid intake

Amount of caffeine intake

Amount of alcohol intake

Amount of urinary output

Time of going to bed

Amount voided at night
(polyuria > 33 per cent of 24-hour volume)

Frequency of leakage

Number of pads per day

Appendix 5
Male Continence Objective Assessment Form

Informed consent:

Abdominal palpation
Distended abdomen (? retention)

Abdominal pain

Perineal and genital examination (in crook lying)
Congenital abnormality

Skin condition (penis, scrotum, perineum and rectal area)

Evidence of infection

Ability to tighten anus

Ability to perform penile retraction and scrotal lift

Leakage on coughing

Ability to prevent leakage on coughing

Dermatomes
S2 lateral buttocks and thigh, posterior calf and plantar heel

S3 upper two-thirds of medial thigh

S4 penis and perineal area

Myotomes
External anal sphincter S2 and S3

Levator ani, ischiococcygeus and bulbocavernosus and bladder S2, S3 and S4

Reflexes
Bulbocavernosus reflex (gentle pressure on the glans penis during
a DRE elicits anal sphincter contraction unless neurological
impairment)

Digital rectal examination

Anterior

◯

Posterior

Sensation of right side of pelvic floor	
Sensation of left side of pelvic floor	
Integrity of right side of anal sphincter	
Integrity of left side of anal sphincter	
Action of puborectalis	
Prostate tested in side lying after training (refer if craggy or hard nodule)	
Pelvic floor strength	0 1 2 3 4 5
Pelvic floor endurance	
Number of repetitions	
Ability to perform fast contractions	

Problems
1
2
3
4

Aims of treatment
1
2
3
4

Treatment

1 _____

2 _____

3 _____

4 _____

Advice

1 _____

2 _____

3 _____

4 _____

Plan

1 _____

2 _____

3 _____

4 _____

Questions for next time

1 _____

2 _____

3 _____

4 _____

Name of physiotherapist _____

Signature

Appendix 6
Pelvic Floor Muscle Exercises for Men

1. In standing

Stand with your feet apart and tighten your pelvic floor muscles as if you were trying to stop the flow of urine and prevent wind escape. If you look in a mirror, you should be able to see the base of your penis move nearer to your abdomen and your testicles raise. Hold the contraction as strongly as you can. Try to avoid holding your breath, pulling in your abdomen or tensing your buttocks.

Perform three maximal contractions in standing in the **morning** holding for ___ seconds.

Perform three maximal contractions in standing in the **evening** holding for ___ seconds.

2. In sitting

Sit on a chair with your knees apart and tighten your pelvic floor muscles as if you were stopping the flow of urine and preventing wind escape. Hold the contraction as strongly as you can. Try to avoid holding your breath, pulling in your abdomen or tensing your buttocks.

Perform three maximal contractions in sitting in the **morning** holding for ___ seconds.

Perform three maximal contractions in sitting in the **evening** holding for ___ seconds.

3. In lying

Lie on your back with your knees bent and your knees apart. Tighten your pelvic floor and hold the contraction as strongly as you can. Try to avoid pulling in your abdomen or tensing your buttocks.

Perform three maximal contractions in lying in the **morning** holding for ___ seconds.

Perform three maximal contractions in lying in the **evening** holding for ___ seconds.

4. While walking

Try lifting up your pelvic floor 50 per cent of maximum when walking.

5. After urinating

After you have voided urine, try tightening your pelvic floor muscles **strongly** to avoid the embarrassing after-dribble.

6. During sexual activity

Try tightening your pelvic floor muscles rhythmically to achieve and maintain penile rigidity during sexual activity. **Slow** thrusting movements generate higher pressures inside the penis.

7. To delay ejaculation

For men with premature ejaculation, try tightening your pelvic floor muscles to delay ejaculation.

Appendix 7
Lifestyle changes

There are a number of ways in which you can change your lifestyle to become generally fitter. These changes may help to improve your penile erections.

Alcohol

Over-consumption of alcohol can lead to erectile difficulties. Try to reduce your daily intake to two units of alcohol a day or less (one pint of beer or two whiskies or two glasses of wine).

0   2   4   6   8   10 units a day

← _____

Smoking

Smoking has been found to adversely affect the circulation. This may produce erectile difficulties. This may be the excuse you need to give up smoking. There are leaflets and support groups which may help you. England Quitline: 08000 002200;
web-site: www.no-smoking-day.org.uk

0   10   20   30   40   50 a day

← _____

General fitness

Men can have erectile difficulties from being unfit as this can put a strain on the heart and the blood pressure. Your fitness may be gradually increased by walking every day and then building up your fitness level by swimming, by sport or by exercising in a gym at least twice a week.

Walking   Exercise 1 x week   Exercise 2 x week   Daily exercise

_____ →

Weight

Obesity can put a strain on the heart and lead to high blood pressure which in turn can affect penile erection. You may find it helpful to join a weight reduction group.

Correct weight   1 stone over   2 stone over   3 stone over   4 stone over
◄───

Cycling

It has been shown that cycling can restrict the circulation to the pelvic floor and the penis. The saddle pressure from prolonged cycling may also damage the nerves to the penis. You may find a change of saddle may help you or taking breaks during your cycle ride.

Not cycling   5 miles   10 miles   20 miles   40 miles
◄───

End of ED/PMD Study/Exit Questionnaire

Name of patient _____ Date _____

1. How is your erectile function now?

Worse	[0]
Same	[1]
Some improvement in rigidity but not fully rigid	[2]
Some improvement in duration but not fully rigid	[3]
Cured	[4]

2. Did you suffer from post micturition dribble before the trial? If so is it now:

Worse	[0]
Same	[1]
Less amount of leakage	[2]
Less amount of leakage and less often	[3]
Cured	[4]

3. Did you suffer from urinary leakage before the trial? If so is it now:

Worse	[0]
Same	[1]
Less leakage	[2]
Less amount of leakage and less often	[3]
Cured	[4]

4. Do you want to continue with your current treatment?

No	[1]
Undecided	[2]
Yes	[3]

5. Tell me how you feel compared to how you were three months ago when you entered the study?

_____

_____

_____

_____

_____

_____

References

Abrams P, Cardozo L, Fall M, Griffiths D, Rosier P, Ulmsten U, van Kerrebroeck P, Victor A, Wein A (2002). The Standardisation of Terminology of Lower Urinary Tract Function: Report from the Standardisation Sub-committee of the International Continence Society. Neurourology and Urodynamics 21: 167–178.

Albaugh J, Lewis JH (1999) Insights into the management of erectile dysfunction: Part I. Urologic Nursing 19(4): 241–247.

Althof SE, Corty EW, Levine SB, Levine F, Burnett AL, McVary K, Stecher V, Seftel AD (1999) EDITS: development of questionnaires for evaluating satisfaction with treatments for erectile dysfunction. Urology 53(4): 793–799.

Amarenco G, Lanoe Y, Perrigot M, Goudal H (1987) Un nouveau syndrome canalaire: la compression du nerf honteux interne dans le canal d'Alcock ou paralysie périnéale du cycliste. Press Med 16: 399.

Andersen KV, Bovim G (1997) Impotence and nerve entrapment in long distance amateur cyclists. Acta Neurology Scandinavia 95(4): 233–240.

Anonymous (1993) A comparison of quality of life with patient reported symptoms and objective findings of men with benign prostatic hyperplasia. The Department of Veterans' Affairs Cooperative Study of Transurethral Resection for Benign Prostatic Hyperplasia. Journal of Urology 150: 1696–1700.

Aydin S, Ercan M, Çaíkurlu T, Taíçi AI, Karaman I, Odabaí O, Yilmaz Y, Aêargün MY, Kara H, Sevin G (1997) Acupuncture and hypnotic suggestions in the treatment of non-organic male sexual dysfunction. Scandinavian Journal of Urology and Nephrology 31: 271–274.

Aytac IA, McKinlay JB, Krane RJ (1999) The likely worldwide increase in erectile dysfunction between 1995 and 2025 and some possible policy consequences. British Journal of Urology International 84: 50–56.

Ballard DJ (1997) Treatment of erectile dysfunction: can pelvic muscle exercises improve sexual function? Journal of Wound Ostomy Continence Nursing 24(5): 255–264.

Baniel J, Israilov S, Shmueli J, Segenreich E, Livne PM (2000) Sexual function in 131 patients with benign prostatic hyperplasia before prostatectomy. European Urology 38(1): 53–58.

Benet AE, Melman A (1995) The epidemiology of erectile dysfunction. Urologic Clinics of North America 22: 699–709.

159

Berger Y (1995) Urodynamic Studies. In Fitzpatrick JM and Krane RJ (eds), The Bladder. London: Churchill Livingstone, 47–70.

Berghmans LCM, Hendriks HJM, Bø K, Hay-Smith EJ, de Bie RA, van Waalwijk van Doorn ESC (1998) Conservative treatment of stress urinary incontinence in women: a systematic review of randomized clinical trials. British Journal of Urology 82: 181–191.

Beutel M (1999) Psychomatic aspects in the diagnosis and treatment of erectile dysfunction. Andrologia 31 (Suppl.1), 37–44.

Bland JM, Altman DG (1996) Measurement error and correlation coefficients. British Medical Journal 313: 41–42.

Blander DS, Sanchez-Ortiz RF, Wein AJ, Broderick GA (2000) Efficacy of sidenafil in erectile dysfunction after radical prostatectomy. International Journal of Impotence Research 12: 165–168.

Bø K, Lilleås F, Talseth T, Hedland H (2001) Dynamic MRI of the pelvic floor muscles in an upright sitting position. Neurourology and Urodynamics 20: 67–174.

Bortolotti A, Parazzini F, Colli E, Landoni M (1997) The epidemiology of erectile dysfunction and its risk factors. International Journal of Andrology 20(6): 323–334.

Bradley WE, Timm GW, Gallagher JM, Johnson BK (1985) New method for continuous measurement of nocturnal penile tumescence and rigidity. Urology 26: 4–9.

Brock GB, Lue TF (1993) Drug-induced male sexual dysfunction: an update. Drug Safety 8(6): 414–426.

Broderick GA (1999) Non-invasive vascular imaging for erectile dysfunction. In CC Carson, RS Kirby, I Goldstein (eds), Textbook of Erectile Dysfunction. Oxford: Isis Medical Media, 233–256.

Brookes ST, Donovan JL, Peters TJ, Abrams P, Neal DE (2002) Sexual dysfunction in men after treatment for lower urinary tract symptoms: evidence from randomised controlled trial. British Medical Journal 324(7345): 1047–1048.

Bruton A (2002) Muscle plasticity: Response to training and detraining. Physiotherapy 88(7): 398–408.

Bullock N (2002) Letter to editor: Initial investigation of choice should be urethral ultrasound. Urology News 6(5): 15.

Bump RC, Hurt WG, Fantl JA, Wyman JF (1991) Assessment of Kegel pelvic muscle exercise performance after brief verbal instruction. American Journal of Obstetrics and Gynecology 165(2): 322–329.

Burgio KL, Stutzman RE, Engel BT (1989) Behavioral training for post-prostatectomy urinary incontinence. The Journal of Urology 141: 303–306.

Byrne P (2002) Making the first consultant post work. Frontline 8(7): 22–23.

Cappelleri JC, Rosen RC (1999) Letter to the Editor. International Journal of Impotence Research 11: 353–354.

Carapeti EA, Kamm MA, Evans BK, Phillips RKS (1999) Topical phenylephrine increases anal sphincter pressure. British Journal of Surgery 86(2): 267–270.

Carter RH, Densley JA, Galley CM, Holland A, Jones LE, Dunn CDR (2001) Factors associated with GP referrals to physiotherapy. British Journal of Therapy and Rehabilitation 8(12): 454–459.

Chadda D (2002) Rewarding excellence in physiotherapy. Frontline 8(11): 9.

Chang, PL, Tsai, LH, Huang, ST, Wang, TM, Hsieh, ML, Tsui, KH (1998) The early effect of pelvic floor muscle exercise after transurethral prostatectomy. Journal of Urology 160(2): 402–405.

Chartered Society of Physiotherapy (1995) Specialisms and specialists. Information Paper No. PA23. London: Chartered Society of Physiotherapy, 1.

Chartered Society of Physiotherapy (1999) Outcome measures. www.csphysio.org.uk London.

Chartered Society of Physiotherapy (2001) Specialisms and specialists: guidance for developing the clinical specialist role. Information Paper No. PA23. London: Chartered Society of Physiotherapy, 1–9.

Chung WS, Sohn JH, Park YY (1999) Is obesity an underlying factor in erectile dysfunction? European Urology 36(1): 68–70.

Claes H, Baert L (1993) Pelvic floor exercise versus surgery in the treatment of impotence. British Journal of Urology 71: 52–57.

Claes H, Bijnens B, Baert L (1996a) The hemodynamic influence of the ischio-cavernosus muscles on erectile function. Journal of Urology 156: 986–990.

Claes HIM, Vandenbroucke HB, Baert LV (1996b) Pelvic floor exercise in the treatment of impotence. The Journal of Urology Supplement 157(4): 786.

Claes H, Van Kampen M, Lysens R, Baert L (1995) Pelvic floor exercises in the treatment of impotence. European Journal of Physical Medicine Rehabilitation 5: 135–140.

Clarys J, Cabri J (1993) Electromyography and the study of sports movements: A review. Journal of Sports Sciences 11: 379–448.

Colpi GM, Negri L, Scroppo FI, Grugnetti C (1994) Perineal floor rehabilitation: a new treatment for venogenic impotence. Journal of Endocrinology Invest 17: 34.

Colpi GM, Negri L, Nappi RE, Chinea B (1999) Perineal floor efficiency in sexually potent and impotent men. International Journal of Impotence Research 11(3): 153–157.

Corcoran M, Smith G, Chisholm GD (1987) Indications for investigation of post-micturition dribble in young adults. British Journal of Urology 59(3): 222–223.

Corty EW, Althof SE, Kurit DM (1996) The reliability and validity of a Sexual Functioning Questionnaire. Journal of Sex and Marital Therapy 22(1): 27–34.

Daines B, Barnes T (1999) Psychotherapy in the treatment of erectile dysfunction. In CC Carson, RS Kirby, I Goldstein (eds), Textbook of Erectile Dysfunction. Oxford: Isis Medical Media, 451–463.

Davies PO (1986) Letter to the Editor. Post-micturition dribbling. Urology 27(3): 288.

DeLancey J (1994) Functional anatomy of the pelvic floor and urinary continence mechanism. In B Schüssler, J Laycock, P Norton, S Stanton (eds), Pelvic Floor Re-education, Principles and Practice. London: Springer-Verlag, 9–21.

Denegar CR, Ball DW (1993) Assessing reliability and precision of measurement: An introduction to intra-class correlation and standard error of measurement. Journal of Sports Rehabilitation 2: 35–42.

Department of Health (2001) The Expert Patient: A New Approach to Chronic Disease Management for the 21st Century. London: The Stationery Office, 1–38.

Derby CA, Araujo AB, Johannes CB, Feldman HA, McKinlay JB (2000a) Measurement of erectile dysfunction in population-based studies: the use of a single question self-assessment in the Massachusetts Male Aging Study. International Journal of Impotence Research 12: 197–204.

Derby CA, Mohr BA, Goldstein I, Feldman HA, Johannes CB, McKinlay JB (2000b) Modifiable risk factors and erectile dysfunction: can lifestyle changes modify risk? Urology 56(2): 302–306.

Derouet H, Nolden W, Jost WH, Osterhage J, Eckert RE, Ziegler M (1998) Treatment of erectile dysfunction by an external ischiocavernosus muscle stimulator. European Urology 34(4): 355–359.

Dinsmore WW, Hodges M, Hargreaves C, Osterloh IH, Smith MD, Rosen RC (1999) Sildenafil citrate (Viagra) in erectile dysfunction: near normalization in men with broad-spectrum erectile dysfunction compared with age-matched healthy control subjects. Urology 53: 800–805.

Dinsmore W, Evans C (1999) ABC of sexual health: Erectile dysfunction. British Medical Journal 318(7180): 387–390.

DiNubile NA (1991) Strength training. Clinical Sports Medicine 10(1): 33–62.

Donaghy ME, Gosling S (1999) Specialisation in physiotherapy: musings on current concepts and possibilities for harmonisation across the European Union. Physical Therapy Review 4: 51–60.

Dorey G (2000) Physiotherapy for the relief of male lower urinary tract symptoms: A Delphi study. Physiotherapy 86(8): 413–426.

Dorey G (2001a) Partners' perspective of erectile dysfunction: literature review. British Journal of Nursing 10(3): 187–195.

Dorey G (2001b) Is smoking a cause of erectile dysfunction? A literature review. British Journal of Nursing 10(7): 455–465.

Dorey G (2001c) Conservative Treatment of Male Urinary Incontinence and Erectile Dysfunction. Ed. G Dorey. London: Whurr.

Dorey G (2001d) Use it or Lose it! Ed. G Dorey. Norfolk: NEEN Healthcare Books.

Dorey G (2002) Prevalence, aetiology and treatment of post-micturition dribble in men: literature review. Physiotherapy 88(4): 219–228.

Dorey G, Swinkels A (2002) Within-day and day-to-day reliability of anal pressure measurements in men. Urologic Nursing 23(3): 214–212.

Durrell S (1996) Expanding the scope of physiotherapy: clinical physiotherapy specialists in consultants' clinics. Manual Therapy 1(4): 210–213.

Fabra M, Porst H (1999) Bulbocavernosus-reflex latencies and pudendal nerve SSEP compared to penile vascular testing in 669 patients with erectile failure and sexual dysfunction. International Journal of Impotence Research 11(3): 167–175.

Feldman HA, Goldstein I, Hatzichristou DG et al. (1994) Impotence and its medical and psychological correlates: results of the Massachusetts Male Ageing Study. Journal of Urology 151: 54–61.

Feneley RCL (1986) Post micturition dribbling. In D Mandelstam (ed.), Incontinence and its Management. London: Croom Helm.

Fishel B, Chen J, Alon M, Zhukovsky G, Matzkin H (2000) The value of testing pudendal nerve conduction in evaluating erectile dysfunction in diabetes. International Journal of Impotence Research 12: 103–105.

Fisher C, Gross J, Zuch J (1965) Cycle of penile erections synchronous with dreaming (REM) sleep. Archives of General Psychiatry 12: 29–45.

Fitts RH, Riley DR, Widrick JJ (2000) Microgravity and skeletal muscle. Journal of Applied Physiology 89: 823–839.

Fletcher EC, Martin RJ (1982) Sexual dysfunction and erectile impotence in chronic obstructive pulmonary disease. Chest 81(4): 413–421.

Frankel SJ, Donovan JL, Peters TJ, Abrams P, Dabhoiwala NF, Osawa D, Tong Long Lin A (1998) Sexual dysfunction in men with lower urinary tract symptoms. Journal of Clinical Epidemiology 51: 677–685.

Frohrib DA, Goldstein I, Peyton TR et al. (1987) Characterization of penile erection states using external computer-based monitoring. Journal of Biomechanical Engineering 109: 110–114.

Furuya S, Ogura H, Tanaka M, Masumori N, Tsukamoto T (1997) Incidence of postmicturition dribble in adult males in their twenties through fifties. Acta Urologica Japonica 43 (6): 407–410 (English Abstract).

Fynes MM, Marshall K, Cassidy M, Behan M, Walsh D, O'Connell PR, O'Herlihy C (1999) A prospective, randomized study comparing the effect of augmented biofeedback with sensory biofeedback alone on fecal incontinence after obstetric trauma. Dis Colon Rectum 42: 753–761.

Glia A, Gylin M, Gullberg K, Lindberg G (1997) Biofeedback retraining in patients with functional constipation and paradoxical puborectalis contraction. Dis Colon Rectum 40: 889–895.

Goldstein I (2000) Oral phentolamine: an alpha-1, alpha-2 adrenergic antagonist for the treatment of erectile dysfunction. International Journal of Impotence Research 12 (Suppl 1): S75–S80.

Goldstein I, Auerbach S, Padma-Nathan H, Rajfer J, Fitch III W, Schmitt L and the Alprostadil Alfadex Study Group (2000) Axial penile rigidity as primary efficacy outcome during multi-institutional in-office dose titration clinical trials with alprostadil alfadex in patients with erectile dysfunction. International Journal of Impotence Research 12: 205–211.

Goldstein I, Lue TF, Padma-Nathan H, Rosen RC, Steers WD, Wicker PA for the Sildenafil Study Group (1998) Oral sildenafil in the treatment of erectile dysfunction. New England Journal of Medicine 338: 1397–1404.

Gosling JA, Dixon JS, Critchley HOD, Thompson SA (1981) A comparative study of the human external sphincter and periurethral levator ani muscle. British Journal of Urology 53: 35–41.

Guyton AC (1986) Textbook of Medical Physiology. Philadelphia, PA: WB Saunders, 1013–1014.

Haslam EJ (1999) Evaluation of pelvic floor muscle assessment, digital, manometric and surface electromyography in females. Unpublished MPhil Thesis. University of Manchester.

Hawton K (1998) Integration of treatments for male erectile dysfunction. The Lancet 351 (9095): 7–8.

Helders PJM, Engelbert RHH, Van der Net J, Gulmans VAM (1999) Physiotherapy quo vadis? Towards an evidence-based, diagnosis-related, functional approach. Advances in Physiotherapy 1: 3–7.

Helgason AR (1997) Prostate cancer treatment and quality of life – a three-level epidemiological approach. University of Stockholm.

Herrington L (1996) EMG biofeedback: What can it actually show? Physiotherapy 82(10): 581–583.

Hicks CM (1995) Research for Pphysiotherapists: Project Design and Analysis. Ed. CM Hicks, 2nd edition. New York: Churchill Livingstone.

Hugonnet CL, Danuser H, Springer JP, Studer UE (1999) Decreased sensitivity in the membranous urethra after orthotopic ileal bladder substitute. Journal of Urology 161: 418–421.

Jackson J, Emerson L, Johnston B, Wilson J, Morales A (1996) Biofeedback: A noninvasive treatment for incontinence after radical prostatectomy. Urologic Nursing 16(2): 50–54.

Jones DA, Round JM (1990) Skeletal Muscle in Health and Disease. Manchester: Manchester University Press, 66–68.

Karpukhin IV, Bogomol'nyi VA (1999) Physical factors in the treatment and rehabilitation of patients with chronic prostatitis complicated by impotence. Vopr Kurortol Fizioter Lech Fiz Kult 2: 25–27.

Kawanishi Y, Yamaguchi K, Kishimoto T, Nakatsuji H, Kojima K, Yamamoto A, Numata A (2000) Simple evaluation of ischiocavernous muscle. International Journal of Impotence Research 12 (Suppl 2): 13.

Keating J, Matyas T (1998) Unreliable inferences from reliable measurements. Australian Physiotherapy 44(1): 5–10.

Kegel A (1948) Progressive resistance exercise in the functional restoration of the perineal muscles. American Journal of Obstetrics and Gynecology 56: 238–248.

Kelley G (1996) Mechanical overload and skeletal muscle fibre hyperplasia: A meta-analysis. Journal of Applied Physiology 81: 1584–1588.

Kho HG, Sweep CG, Chen X, Rabsztyn PR, Meuleman EJ (1999) The use of acupuncture in the treatment of erectile dysfunction. International Journal of Impotence Research 11(1): 41–46.

Kirby R, Carson C, Goldstein I (1999) Anatomy, physiology and pathophysiology. In R Kirby (ed), Erectile Dysfunction: A Clinical Guide. Oxford: Isis Medical Media, 11–28.

Kondo A, Lin TL, Nordling J, Siroky M, Tammela T (2002) Conservative Management in men. In P Abrams, L Cardozo, S Khoury, A Wein (eds), Incontinence. Second International Consultation on Incontinence, 2nd edition. Plymouth: Plymbridge Distributors, 553–569.

Koskimäki J, Makama M, Huhtala H, Tammela TLJ (1998) Prevalence of lower urinary tract symptoms in Finnish men: a population-based study. British Journal of Urology 81: 364–369.

Krane R, Brock G, Eardley I, Fourcroy J, Giuliano F, Hutter A, Teloken C, Vickers M (2000) Oral non-endocrine treatment. In A Jardin, G Wagner, S Khoury, F Giuliano, H Padma-Nathan, R Rosen (eds), Erectile Dysfunction. Plymouth: Plymbridge, 241–304.

Krane RJ, Goldstein I, Saenz De Tejada I (1989) Medical progress: impotence. New England Journal of Medicine 321: 1648–1659.

Kunelius P, Lukkarinen O (1999) Intracavernosus self-injection of prostaglandin E1 in the treatment of erectile dysfunction. International Journal of Impotence Research 11: 21–24.

La Pera G, Nicastro A (1996) A new treatment for premature ejaculation: the rehabilitation of the pelvic floor. Journal of Sex and Marital Therapy 22(1): 22–26.

Lavoisier P, Courtois F, Barres D, Blanchard M (1986) Correlation between intracavernous pressure and contraction of the ischiocavernosus muscle in man. Journal of Urology 136: 936–939.

Lavoisier P, Proulx J, Courtois F, De Carufel F, Durand L (1988) Relationship between perineal muscle contractions, penile tumescence, and penile rigidity during nocturnal erections. Journal of Urology 139: 176–179.

Lavoisier P, Schmidt M, Alaoui R (1992) Intracavernous pressure increases and perineal muscle contractions in response to pressure stimulation of the glans penis. International Journal of Impotence Research 4: 157.

Laycock J (1994a) Clinical evaluation of the pelvic floor. In Shussler B, Laycock J, Norton P, Stanton S (eds), Pelvic Floor Re-education. Principle and Practice. London: Springer-Verlag, 42–48.

Laycock J (1994b) Female pelvic floor assessment: the Laycock ring of continence. Journal of the National Women's Health Group, Australian Physiotherapy Association 13: 40–51.

Laycock J, Irvine L, Emery S (1999) General principles of conservative treatment. In M Lucas, S Emery, J Benyon (eds), Incontinence. Oxford: Blackwell Science, 67–86.

Levine LA, Lenting EL (1999) Use of nocturnal penile tumescence and rigidity in the evaluation of male erectile dysfunction. Urologic Clinics of North America 22: 775–788.

Lewis RW, Mills TM (1999) Risk factors for impotence. In CC Carson, RS Kirby and I Goldstein (eds), Textbook of Erectile Dysfunction. Oxford: Isis Medical Media, 141–148.

Likert RA (1952) A technique for the development of attitude scales. Educational and Psychological Measurement 12: 313–315.

Lombardi G (1999) Reprogrammation sensitivo mortice dans le syndrome de l'éjaculation prematée. Abstract in Conference proceedings. Premières recontres méditérranéennes d'actualités thérapeutiques réhabilitatives sur les dysfonctions du plancher pelvien. Marseilles, 19, 20, 21 November.

Lording DW, McMahon CG, Conaglen JV, Earle C, Gillman MP, Tulloch AGS (2000) Partners of affected men: attitudes to erectile dysfunction. International Journal of Impotence Research. Proceedings of the Seventh Biennial Asia-Pacific Meeting on Impotence. 26–30 October 1999, Tokyo, 12(2): S16.

Lowentritt BH, Scardino PT, Miles BJ, Orejuela FJ, Schatte EC, Slawin KM, Elliott SP, Kim ED (1999) Sildenafil citrate after radical prostatectomy. Journal of Urology 1625(5): 1614.

Lucas M, Emery S, Benyon J (1999) Specialist investigations. In M Lucas, S Emery, J Benyon (eds), Incontinence. Oxford: Blackwell Science, 67–86.

MacDonagh R, Ewings P, Porter T (2002) The effect of erectile dysfunction on quality of life: Psychometric testing of a new quality of life measure for patients with erectile dysfunction. Journal of Urology 167: 212–217.

Macfarlane GJ, Botto H, Sagnier P, Teillac P, Richard F, Boyle P (1996) The relationship between sexual life and urinary condition in the French community. Journal of Clinical Epidemiology 49(10): 1171–1176.

Malmsten UGH, Milsom I, Molander U, Norlen LJ (1997) Urinary incontinence and lower urinary tract symptoms: an epidemiological study of men aged 45 to 99 years. Journal of Urology 158: 1733–1737.

Mamberti-Dias A, Bonierbale-Branchereau M (1991) Therapy for dysfunctioning erections: four years later, how do things stand? Sexologique 1: 24–25.

Mamberti-Dias A, Vasavada SP, Bourcier AP (1999) Pelvic floor dysfunction: investigations and conservative treatment. Casa Editrice Scientifica Internationale, 303–310.

Marzio L, Ciccaglione FA, Falcucci M, Malatesta MG, Grossi L, Travaglini N, Guerri S (1998) Relationship between anal canal diameter and pressure evaluated simultaneously by endosonography and manometry in normal subjects. International Journal of Colorectal Disease 13: 21–26.

Mattiasson A, Djurhuus JC, Fonda D, Lose G, Nordling J, Stöhrer M (1998) Standardization of outcome studies in patients with lower urinary tract dysfunction. Neurourology and Urodynamics 17: 249–253.

Meehan JP, Goldstein AMB (1983) High pressure within corpus cavernosum in man during erection. Its probable mechanism. Urology 21: 385.

Michal V, Simana J, Rehak J, Masim J (1983) Haemodynamics of erection in man. Physiologia Bohemoslovaca 32: 497.

Mikhailidis DP, Ganotakis ES, Papadakis JA, Jeremy JY (1998) Smoking and urological disease. Journal of Research in Social Health 118(4): 210–212.

Miller J, Ashton-Miller JA, DeLancey JOL (1996) The Knack: use of precisely-timed pelvic muscle contraction can reduce leakage in SUI. Neurourology and Urodynamics 15(4): 392–393.

Millard RJ (1989) After-dribble. In RJ Millard (ed), Bladder Control – A Simple Self-help Guide. New South Wales: William and Wilkins and Associates 89–90.

Moncada Iribarren I, Sáenz de Tejada I (1999) Vascular physiology of penile erection. In CC Carson, RS Kirby, I Goldstein (eds), Textbook of Erectile Dysfunction. Oxford: Isis Medical Media 51–57.

Moore A, McQuay HJ (2002) What is an NNT? www.evidence-based-medicine.co.uk 1(1): 1–4.

Moore KN, Griffiths DJ, Hughton A (1999) A randomised controlled trial comparing pelvic muscle exercises with pelvic muscle exercises plus electrical stimulation for the treatment of post-prostatectomy urinary incontinence. British Journal of Urology 83: 57–65.

Morris J (2002) Current issues of accountability in physiotherapy and higher education. Physiotherapy 88(6): 354–363.

National Institutes of Health Consensus Development Panel on Impotence (1993) Impotence. Journal of the American Medical Association 270: 83–90.

Nehra A, Pryor J, Althof SE et al. (2002) Overview consensus statement. Second International Conference on Management of Erectile Dysfunction: New perspectives on treatment. International Journal of Impotence Research 14 (Suppl 1) S1–S5.

Norton C, Hosker G, Brazzelli M (2000) Biofeedback and/or sphincter exercises for the treatment of faecal incontinence in adults. The Cochrane Library (Issue 4) 1–49.

O'Leary MP, Fowler FJ, Lenderking WR, Barber B, Sagnier PP, Guess HA, Barry MJ (1995) A brief male sexual function inventory for urology. Urology 46: 697–706.

Osterloh I, Eardley I, Carson C, Padma-Nathan H (1999) Sildenafil: a selective phosphodiesterase (PDE)5 inhibitor in the treatment of erectile dysfunction (ED) In CC Carson, RS Kirby and I Goldstein (eds), Textbook of Erectile Dysfunction. Oxford: Isis Medical Media 285–308.

Paterson J, Pinnock CB, Marshall, VR (1997) Pelvic floor exercises as a treatment for post-micturition dribble. British Journal of Urology 79: 892–897.

Porru D, Campus G, Caria A, Madeddu G, Cucchi A, Rovereto B, Scarpa RM, Pili P, Usai E (2001) Impact of early pelvic floor rehabilitation after transurethral resection of the prostate. Neurourology and Urodynamics 20: 53–59.

Prostate Trials Office (2000) PROstate Trials Office sex instrument (PROTOsex). www.proto.org. London.

Recommendations of the First International Consultation on Erectile Dysfunction (2000) In A Jardin, G Wagner, S Khoury, F Giuliano, H Padma-Nathan, R Rosen (eds), Erectile Dysfunction. Plymouth: Plymbridge Distributors 711–726.

Rendell MS, Rajfer J, Wicker PA, Smith MD (1999) Sildenfil for treatment of erectile dysfunction in men with diabetes: a randomized controlled trial. Journal of the American Medical Association 281(5): 421–426.

Research Governance Framework for Health and Social Care (2001) Research and Development Information for Health and Social Care. London: Department of Health, www.researchinformation.nhs.uk/main/governance.htm.

Richardson B (1993) Practice, research and education: What is the link? Physiotherapy 79: 317–322.

Rosen MP, Greenfield AJ, Walker TG, Grant P, Dubrow J, Bettmann MA, Fried LE, Goldstein I (1991) Cigarette smoking: an independent risk factor for atherosclerosis in the hypogastric-cavernous arterial bed of men with arteriogenic impotence. Journal of Urology 145(4): 759–763.

Rosen RC, Cappelleri JC, Gendrano III N (2002) The International Index of Erectile Function (IIEF): a state-of-the-science review. International Journal of Impotence Research 14: 226–244.

Rosen RC, Cappelleri JC, Smith MD, Lipsky J, Peña BM (1999a) Development and evaluation of an abridged, 5-item version of the International Index of Erectile Function (IIEF-5) as a diagnostic tool for erectile dysfunction. International Journal of Impotence Research 11(6): 319–326.

Rosen R, Padma-Nathan H, Goldstein I (1999b) Process of care model for the management of erectile dysfunction in the primary care setting. In CC Carson, RS Kirby and I Goldstein (eds), Textbook of Erectile Dysfunction. Oxford: Isis Medical Media, 497–506.

Rosen RC, Riley A, Wagner G, Osterloh IH, Kirkpatrick J, Mishra A (1997) The International Index of Erectile Function (IIEF): a multidimensional scale for assessment of erectile dysfunction. Urology 49: 822–830.

Sackett DL (1986) How are we to determine whether dietary interventions do more good than harm to hypertensive patients? Canadian Journal of Physiology and Pharmacology 64(6): 781–783.

Sale D (1992) Neural adaptation to strength training. In P Komi (ed), Strength and Power in Sport. Oxford: Blackwell Scientific, chapter 9A.

Savoye G, Leroi AM, Denis P, Michot F (2000) Manometric assessment of an artificial bowel sphincter. British Journal of Surgery 87(5): 586–589.

Schouman M, Lacroix P (1991) Apport de la ré-éducation pelvi-périnéale au traitement des fuites veino-caverneuses. Ann Urologique 25: 92–93.

Schwarzer U, Sommer F, Klotz T, Cremer C, Engelmann U (2002) Cycling and penile oxygen pressure: the type of saddle matters. European Urology 41(2): 139–143.

Shafik A (1996) Extrapelvic cavernous nerve stimulation in erectile dysfunction. Human study. Andrologia 28(3): 151–156.

Shafik A (1999) The physioanatomic entirety of the external anal sphincter with the bulbocavernosus muscle: a new concept. Arch Androl 42: 45–54.

Shafik A (2000) The role of the levator ani muscle in evacuation, sexual performance and pelvic floor disorders. International Urogynecology Journal 11(6): 361–376.

Shafik A, El-Sibai O (2000a) Mechanism of ejection during ejaculation: identification of a urethrocavernosus reflex. Archives of Andrology 44 (1): 77–83.

Shafik A, El-Sibai O (2000b) The anocavernosal erectile dysfunction syndrome II Anal fissure and erectile dysfunction. International Journal of Impotence Research 12: 279–283.

Shah, PJR (1994) The assessment of patients with a view to urodynamics. In AR Mundy, TP Stephenson, A Wein (eds), Urodynamics, Principles, Practice and Application. Edinburgh: Churchill Livingstone 59.

Slob AK, Cornelissen S, Dohle GR, Gijs L, van der Werff ten Bosch JJ (2002) The limited practical value of color Doppler sonography in the differential diagnosis of men with erectile dysfunction. International Journal of Impotence Research 14: 201–203.

Stephenson TP, Farrar DJ (1977) Urodynamic study of 15 patients with postmicturition dribble. Urology 9(4): 404–406.

Stewart M (1998) Advanced practice in physiotherapy. Physiotherapy 84(4): 184–186.

Stief CG (2002) Is there a common pathophysiology of erectile dysfunction and how does this relate to new pharmacotherapies? International Journal of Impotence Research 14 (Suppl 1) S11–S16.

Stief CG, Weller E, Noack T, Djamilian, MH, Meschi M, Truss M, Jonas U (1996) Functional electromyostimulation of the penile corpus cavernosum (FEMCC). Initial results of a new therapeutic option of erectile dysfunction. Urologe A 35(4): 321–325.

Strasser H, Klauser A, Helweg G, Frauscher F, Pallwein G, Bartsch G (2001) Three-dimensional transrectal ultrasound of the male urethral rhabdosphincter. Second International Consultation on Incontinence, Paris (abstract).

Sueppel C, Kreder K, See W (2001) Improved continence outcomes with preoperative pelvic floor muscle strengthening exercises. Urologic Nursing 21(3): 201–210.

Tan HM, Moh CLC, Mendoza JB, Gana Jr. T, Albano GJ, De la Cruz R, Chye PLH, Sam CCW for the ASSESS-1 Study Group (2000) Asian sildenafil efficacy and safety study (ASSESS-1): a double-blind, placebo controlled, flexible dose study of oral sildenafil in Malaysian, Singaporean, and Filipino men with erectile dysfunction. The Assess-1 study group. Urology 56: 635–640.

Tan RS, Philip PS (1999) Perceptions of and risk factors for andropause. Archives of Andrology 43(3): 227–233.

Timm G (1999) Editorial comment. International Journal of Impotence Research 11(6): 327–339.

Turner LA, Althof SE, Levine SB et al (1992) Twelve month comparison of two treatments for erectile dysfunction: self-injection versus external vacuum devices. Urology 39:139–144.

Udelson D, Park K, Sadeghi-Najed H, Salimpour P, Krane RJ, Goldstein I (1999) Axial penile buckling forces vs Rigiscan™ radial rigidity as a function of intra-cavernosal pressure: why Rigiscan™ does not predict functional erections in individual patients. International Journal of Impotence Research 11: 327–339.

Van Kampen M, De Weerdt W, Claes H, Feys H, De Maeyer M, Van Poppel H, Baert L (1998) Contribution of the pelvic floor muscles exercises in the treatment of impotence. PhD thesis, Katholieke Universiteit Leuven, Belgium.

Van Kampen M, De Weerdt W, Van Poppel H, De Ridder D, Feys H, Baert L (2000) Effect of pelvic floor re-education on duration and degree of incontinence after radical prostatectomy: a randomised controlled trial. The Lancet 355(9198): 98–102.

Vereecken RL, Puers B, Van Mulders J (1982) Spectral analysis of perineal muscles EMG. Electromyographic Clinical Neurophysiology 22: 321–326.

Vereecken RL, Verduyn H (1970) The electrical activity of the paraurethral and perineal muscles in normal and pathological conditions. British Journal of Urology 42: 457–463.

Vodušek D (1994) Electrophysiology. In B Schüssler, J Laycock, P Norton, S Stanton (eds), Pelvic Floor Re-education: Principles and Practice. London: Springer Verlag, 83–97.

Wagner G, The Lygon Arms Group: Claes H, Costa P, Cricelli C, De Boer J, Debruyne FMJ, Dean J, Dinsmore WW, Fitzpatrick JM, Ralph DJ, Hackett GI, Heaton JP, Hatzichristou DG, Mendive J, Meuleman EJ, Mirone V, Montorsi F,

Raineri F, Schulman CC, Stief CG, Von Keitz AT, Wright PJ (2002) A shared care approach to the management of erectile dysfunction in the community. International Journal of Impotence Research 14: 189–194.

Wagner SG, Pfeifer A, Cranfield TL, Craik RL (1994) The effects of ageing on muscle strength and function: a review of the literature. Physiotherapy and Practice 10(1): 9–16.

Wagner TH, Patrick DL, McKenna SP, Froese PS (1996) Cross-cultural development of a quality of life measure for men with erection difficulties. Quality of Life Research 5: 443–449.

Wespes E, Nogueira MC, Herbaut AG, Caufriez M, Schulman CC (1990) Role of the bulbocavernosus muscles on the mechanism of human erection. European Urology 18: 45–48.

Wille S, Mills RD, Studer UE (2000) Absence of urethral post-void milking: an additional cause for incontinence after radical prostatectomy? European Urology 37: 665–669.

Wyllie MG (2000) Clinical trials design: protocols and endpoints. International Journal of Impotence Research 12 (Suppl 4) S53–S58.

Wyndaele JJ, Van Eetvelde B (1996) Reproducibility of digital testing of the pelvic floor muscles in men. Archives of Physical Medicine and Rehabilitation 77(11): 1179–1181.

Yang CC, Bradley WE (1999) Somatic innervation of the human bulbocavernosus muscle. Clinical Neurophysiology 110(3): 412–418.

Yang CC, Bradley WE (2000) Reflex innervation of the bulbocavernosus muscle. British Journal of Urology International 85(7): 857–863.

Index